Not your ordinary doctor

JIM LEAVESLEY

Not
your ordinary doctor

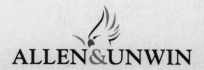
ALLEN&UNWIN

First published in 2010

Allen & Unwin
83 Alexander Street
Crows Nest NSW 2065
Australia
Phone: (61 2) 8425 0100
Fax: (61 2) 9906 2218
Email: info@allenandunwin.com
Web: www.allenandunwin.com

Cataloguing-in-Publication details are available
from the National Library of Australia
www.librariesaustralia.nla.gov.au

ISBN 978 1 74237 330 0

Internal images are courtesy of Photolibrary
Set in 11/15.5 pt Goudy Oldstyle by Post Pre-press Group, Australia
Printed in Australia by McPherson's Printing Group

10 9 8 7 6 5 4 3 2 1

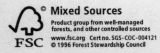

Mixed Sources
Product group from well-managed
forests, and other controlled sources
www.fsc.org Cert no. SGS-COC-004121
© 1996 Forest Stewardship Council

The paper in this book is FSC certified.
FSC promotes environmentally responsible,
socially beneficial and economically viable
management of the world's forests.

This book is dedicated to Robyn Williams and Brigitte Seega of the ABC Radio National Science Unit for all their help and encouragement in my writing and broadcasting over the last 28 years

Contents

PART III   Doctors who have been adventurers, inventors, athletes or politicians

PART IV   Doctors who have been criminals

Preface

Throughout history, from the earliest times, doctors have worked and prospered outside the profession for which they were originally trained. They have been consulted or relied upon by national leaders, dictators or royalty, been the cause of court jealousies or intrigues, and the conveyers of bad or good news—more often the former. Some have even committed high treason by, say, sharing the bed of a monarch. More commonly their interest away from clinical medicine has been of a more artistic nature, finding fame as authors, musicians or actors. Many have been world-famous sportsmen or sportswomen, adventurers or inventors. Criminals—especially murderers—have appeared among their ranks.

In this book I want to look at some well-known examples of such 'medical truants'. After a brief look at some medical personnel from ancient times, our noteworthy physicians are grouped under four main headings, and the genesis of their fame examined. Their actual medical expertise will usually get a mention, but it is their extracurricular activities that will be the main interest.

Keeping this book within reasonable bounds has left me with two main regrets. First, very few women are included: female doctors did not appear on the medical scene until the latter part of the nineteenth century, and most of the doctors examined in this book precede this era. The second regret is that many deserving examples—at least another book's worth—have been omitted for reasons of space. Perhaps the most notable omission is the case of Dr Harold Shipman, the most notorious medical murderer of recent times. As his well-known story is fresh in our memories and has been so well recorded, I have left its recounting to those who have told it already. But I hope those people who have been examined, some in more detail than others but all with an interesting 'other life', are enough to provide a fascinating glimpse of medical roads less travelled.

Acknowledgements

I am delighted to acknowledge the examples suggested by, and help received from, many people. For their input of ideas and help in tracking down the background of the subjects, I am most grateful.

Leading the field in thanks must be Ms Carol Newton-Smith and Mr Simon Lewis, respectively Chief Librarian and Senior Reference Librarian at the University of Western Australia Medical and Dental Library. They have been tireless in bringing up obscure references and suggesting candidates. I am also grateful to Dr Kerri Parnell, Editor of the medical newspaper *Australian Doctor*, for allowing me to use some of the material I have written for the publication over the last twenty years, and also for the interest of her resourceful staff, especially Geraldine Kurukchi and Shahiron Sahari. Also my cousin, Jim Leavesley, who lives in Staffordshire, England, and who visited the nearby town of Rugeley to obtain first-hand material on the murderer Dr William Palmer. Sir Barry Jackson, a past president of the Royal College of Surgeons of England and former Sergeant Surgeon to Queen Elizabeth II, provided invaluable information about the history of the medical establishment in the royal household. Emeritus Professor Sol Encel was consulted on medically qualified female politicians. Dr Ric Charlesworth informed me about his sporting background and 'handedness'. Ms Carole Rutter provided details of a number of medical criminals. A special thanks goes to Stuart Neal, Consultant Publisher at Allen & Unwin, a man full of ideas who first floated the concept of the book, and who has been most supportive and patient throughout the project. Also to Jo Lyons, the helpful editor of the book, and Katri Hilden, the tireless copyeditor. Last, but by no means least in the thank-you list, is my wife, Margaret. Writing a book is not a spectator sport; it is a solitary occupation, which in my case was made more bearable and enjoyable by her regularly plying me with coffee, snacks and snippets of news from the outside world. As always, she was a great support.

Finally, it will be noted that the book is dedicated to Robyn Williams and Brigitte Seega of the ABC's Radio National Science Unit. In January 1982 I was invited to record four programs to do with the medical history of four famous people, which I had submitted to what was then called *The Body Program*; since 1984 it has been known as *Ockham's Razor*. Having once tried me out, I was invited back and under the guidance of Robyn as presenter and Brigitte as producer have been a regular contributor ever since. Over the years they encouraged me with good humour and enthusiasm to continue, and I am eternally grateful for their belief in my slightly offbeat and irreverent medical essays; or maybe it is my North of England accent which has made them popular. Out of these numerous broadcasts a number of books have been published; this is my eleventh and contains some of my *Ockham's* material.

But for Robyn and Brigitte they would probably have never seen the light of day. I am eternally grateful to them for showing me the way.

Jim Leavesley
Margaret River
Western Australia
July 2010

1

In the beginning

By way of introduction to the expanded medical talent to come, let us briefly look at a few of the very early doctors who were associated with rulers or national leaders in antiquity. On the whole little is known about ancient Egyptian and Greek medical practitioners, but the following four stand out.

Sekhet'enanach

The earliest name in medical history is that of Sekhet'enanach, who lived about 3000 BC and was chief physician to one of the Pharaohs. His tomb has been discovered and in it is a stone statue of the man, dressed in a leopard skin and carrying two sceptres. It is recorded of the physician that 'he healed the king's nostrils'. An odd claim to fame, but it seems that rather than accept a fee, he requested that his likeness be fashioned in stone, that the monarch's nose problem, whatever it was, be recorded for posterity, and that his statue should be set up in his tomb when he died. His wishes were respected and as a result, 5000 years later, he is the first physician in world history to be known to us by name.

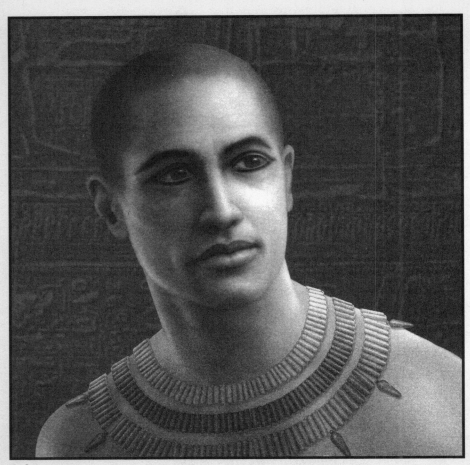

Imhotep

Imhotep

There is, however, a more famous medical man from that early Egyptian era whose life is much better documented. His name was Imhotep and he lived between about 2980 and 2900 BC. The doctor was the medical adviser and grand vizier to King Djoser, second king of the Third Dynasty. A vizier was a leading court official or bureaucrat who presided over various state departments.

A number of statues of Imhotep are still extant; several stand in the Wellcome Historical Medical Museum and British Museum in London. Oddly, he was better known as an architect and vizier to the Pharaoh than as a doctor, though for long after his death he was worshipped first as a demigod, and then the god of medicine. That accolade lasted until well into the Christian era, and numerous of his 'sayings' were preserved among contemporary Egyptian wisdom. Really, on account of his antiquity, it should be Imhotep, rather than the well-known Hippocrates (? 460–377 BC), who should be regarded as the 'father of medicine'. (Regrettably, Hippocrates himself does not qualify for a place in this chapter as he was a pure physician who devoted himself to medicine.)

Apart from his medical and vizier positions, Imhotep was high priest at Heliopolis, a city near the apex of the Nile delta and a centre of sun worship; he was also an astrologer, sage and, most famously, the architect of the Step Pyramid of Saqqarah, the oldest surviving stone building in the world. It still stands near Memphis, the ancient centre of Lower (northern) Egypt on the

Nile, for all to see and marvel over. The building comprises six steps and stands about 60 metres high.

The name Imhotep means 'he who cometh in peace', and he was held in such high esteem that at least three temples were built in his honour, one each at Memphis, Thebes and the island of Philae. Only the temple on Philae, far up the Nile in Upper (southern) Egypt, remains, but even that has now been submerged under the waters of the Aswan Dam.

Fittingly, the ancient polymath was buried near Memphis, but his tomb has not been found.

Glaucias

One of the great relationships in history was that between Alexander the Great—a charismatic, outgoing man and one of the ancient world's greatest leaders—and his First Lieutenant and gay lover, Hephaestion.

Both were born in Macedonia; Alexander in 356 BC, and his trusty Hephaestion probably the same year. As young men, both were tutored by the famed philosopher, Aristotle. Alexander had a wife—Roxana, daughter of Oxyartes, a Bactrian nobleman—and in the spring of 324 BC Hephaestion married her sister, thus tightening the bond between the two men by becoming brothers-in-law. Little is known about Hephaestion's other relationships, but the one with his commander was close and enduring.

In that same year, 324 BC, the Greek army travelled to the city of Ecbatana, in what is now Syria. They arrived in autumn, whereupon Hephaestion fell ill with a fever. It ran for seven days, and though it may have been the common local misery, malaria, in the light of subsequent events it was probably typhoid fever. He was treated by his commander's doctor, Glaucias. Regrettably, little is known about this important medical figure of the ancient world, except that he was, apparently, a very competent physician. This, however, would not save him from a terrible fate, becoming one of the first doctors in history to be murdered for medical 'incompetence'.

Doubtless in more 'primitive' communities, the local medicine man or shaman may have been strangled by bereaved relatives for, say, a botched trephining of the skull with subsequent death of the patient, but records of such events were never kept. The death of Glaucias, however, was recorded for us by the scribes of the time. Several centuries later, Glaucias's life underwent a more exacting examination by the Greek historian and philosopher Arrian, who lived from about 95 to 175 AD, but regrettably, given this large lapse in time, much of what he wrote about the doctor was probably hearsay.

It seems that after a week of feeling ill, Hephaestion began to feel much better, but the medical advice from Glaucias was to continue resting and to take a light diet. The good doctor and Alexander then left Hephaestian to rest and went off to the theatre, whereupon the patient disobeyed orders by getting up and eating a hearty meal and imbibing alcohol. Fairly quickly afterwards he fell ill with severe stomach pains and died.

Why this happened is not certain, but if his illness had been due to typhoid and not some other endemic tropical disease, the solid food he consumed could have perforated any existing bowel ulcerations—the so-called Peyer's patches, a well-known and sometimes fatal feature of typhoid fever. Another possibility was that his food may have been poisoned by a jealous rival.

Whatever the cause, Hephaestion's death had a profound effect on Alexander the Great, whose grief was described several centuries later by Plutarch (c. 45–120 AD) as 'being uncontrollable'. Alexander stormed and raged, but, of course, to no avail. He then sank into a deep depression and ordered several acts of mourning to be carried out, such as cutting his own hair short, and docking the tails and manes of his horses, the pride of both animals and their keepers. He ordered the Temple of Asclepius at Ecbatana to be razed to the ground, even though he had worshipped there. He banned ceremonial flutes and every other type of music and lay sleeping on top of his erstwhile lover's dead body, which in the ambient climate would have been none too inviting a bed after a day or two. In the end he had to be forcibly dragged away from his noisome mattress. He did not eat for two days. The depth of his mourning was obviously of a pathological degree, made worse by his position of absolute power, which allowed him to carry on such excesses without questions being asked or advice sought.

But his worst excess was that, in a moment of unalloyed grief, he had the attending doctor, Glaucias, killed for incompetence, even though the faithful physician had given specific instructions about diet and drinking alcohol to his patient and was guiltless of the untimely death. It is thought Glaucias was executed by crucifixion, a particularly painful and lingering way to die. Whatever the method chosen, Glaucias certainly got a raw deal.

Unlike Glaucias, Hephaestion was given a magnificent funeral: Alexander himself drove the funeral cart part of the way back to Babylon, where funeral games involving 3000 competitors were held in the dead man's honour. As a final tribute, on the day of the actual funeral orders were given to extinguish the sacred flame in the Temple—an observance normally reserved for the death of a king.

Amid the excesses of grief surrounding the lover's death, the hapless doctor would not in fact be forgotten. Alexander and his Macedonian henchmen may have considered him dead and buried, but to the medical historian Glaucias is now remembered as our first medical martyr.

Aristotle

Aristotle (384–322 BC) from Stagira in Thrace was, of course, one of Ancient Greece's most famous philosophers. His father was a doctor and though he himself had no formal medical training, his keen interest and work in biology—especially botany—was of inestimable value in medical practice, in which he dabbled. Besides his philosophising, Aristotle was a scientific genius who had a highly significant role in contemporary medical experimentation.

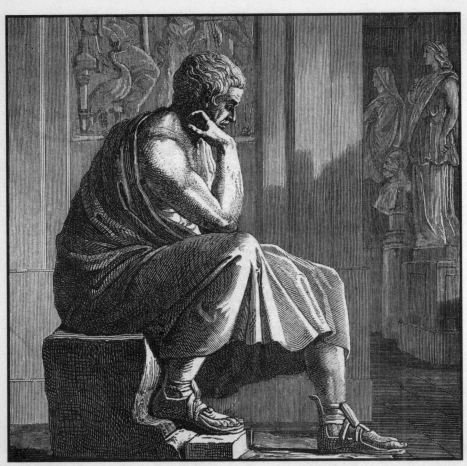

Aristotle

As an adult Aristotle lived in Athens, where he was a pupil of Plato. They argued about metaphysics, ethics, politics and the scientific method; Aristotle later became tutor to Philip of Macedonia's son, Alexander the Great, whose treatment of Dr Glaucias some years later was, as we have seen, hardly Aristotelian in its execution, so to speak.

The philosopher-cum-doctor investigated the natural world and laid the foundations of comparative anatomy and embryology. He was the first to systematically use dissection of animals as a grounding for medical theories. He dissected innumerable animals, especially fish, and his descriptions and classifications remained sound until recently. Because he did not dissect humans, some of his observations regarding the human state were erroneous. For instance, he thought the human heart had three chambers; it has four. And he did not distinguish between veins and arteries.

Aristotle followed Hippocrates in believing the body possessed four fundamental qualities—the hot and the cold, the dry and the wet—and that it was composed of four 'humours': blood, phlegm, yellow bile and black bile. Any disturbance in their relationship to each other was the trigger that led to disease. His work on the chick within the egg, where he observed the first beatings of the heart, were the first steps in the study of embryology.

Though primarily a philosopher at heart, Aristotle was a remarkable polymath, and his place in the field of medicine is assured.

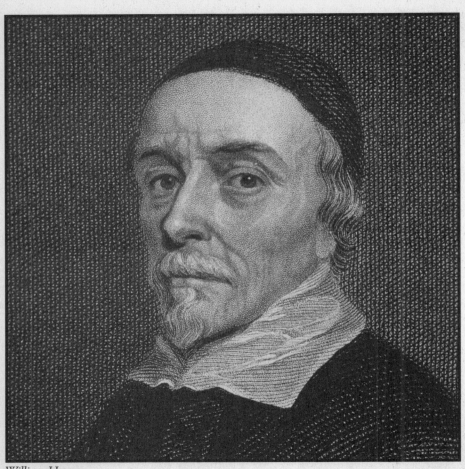

William Harvey

PART I

Doctors to royalty and national leaders

2

Two royal doctors who came to a sticky end

Dr Ruy Lopez (c. 1525–1594)

A Portuguese doctor of Jewish background, Ruy Lopez was driven from his country by the Spanish Inquisition and settled in London at the beginning of Queen Elizabeth I's reign in 1558. There he set up as a general practitioner, as we would call it nowadays. He prospered and became a physician at the prestigious St Bartholomew's Hospital, already then 400 years old (and still going strong). As his deserved reputation grew, he was sought as a medical adviser to the aristocracy and well-to-do, until he rose to the country's top job in 1575 as Physician-in-Chief to the 'Virgin Queen' herself. For a sixteenth-century doctor, life did not come much better than that.

Despite the predictable racial mutterings and murmurings against a foreigner attaining such an elevated position, and professional rivalry claiming he owed his advancement more to flattery than medical skill, Lopez flourished, displaying all the outward trappings of wealth and fame, safely ensconced in the favour of the monarch. By October 1593, the prosperous doctor had a son at the prestigious and expensive Winchester School (which is still going strong too), and a house in trendy Holborn, London.

But the political climate of the day was treacherous. At the time, Spain and Portugal were England's sworn enemies and there was much intrigue and plotting within England and the Continent by spies and double agents. The leader of the anti-Spanish and Portuguese faction in England was the Earl of Essex, and it came to his notice that a certain Portuguese gentleman, Esteban Ferreira, was living in Lopez's house and had offered his services to Spain. The Earl told the Queen, and Ferreira was accordingly seized and put in custody without charges being laid.

When Lopez heard of this outrage, he went to the Queen and begged for the release of his countryman, observing that if released he could be employed to 'work a peace between the two kingdoms'. This did not sit well with Her Majesty, so enigmatically, and without thinking it through, he added, 'If your Majesty does not desire that course, might not the deceiver be deceived'. Elizabeth was not sure what he meant by this, but decided he was certainly taking a liberty. The doctor, perceiving he had not made a good impression, bowed himself out of the room. (We know this thanks to Francis Bacon, who recorded it at the time.)

Shortly afterwards and after a second tip-off, another visiting Portuguese was arrested while carrying a suspicious letter. When apprehended he was incautious enough to ask that news of his arrest be conveyed to Lopez, thus implicating the good doctor. Later he was shown the 'rack' and other torture instruments in the Tower of London, whereupon his courage forsook him and he immediately spilled the beans about the letter's treasonous content.

At about the same time, the imprisoned Ferreira had managed to smuggle out an incriminating note to Dr Lopez about this third party. Lopez replied and both letters were seized. When interviewed Ferreira confessed, gratuitously adding that Lopez had been in the pay of Spain for years and was a principal foreign agent. Doubtless some kind of physical enforcement was involved to extract this information.

So it came to pass that on 1 January 1594 the Queen's doctor, Ruy Lopez, was arrested. His house was searched, but nothing incriminating was found. He was interviewed by the statesman Robert Cecil, who concluded there was nothing in it and that the Earl of Essex was merely stirring up a hornet's nest in his anti-Spanish fervour, seeing spies under every bed. Cecil informed the Queen that as regards Doctor Lopez, all was well. The displeased Elizabeth called in the 28-year-old Earl and told him he was 'a rash and temerarious youth'.

The Earl left the royal presence with what good grace he could muster, determined to bring Dr Lopez to justice, knowing that anyone accused of High Treason was virtually never acquitted, for reasons of expediency, rather than justice. The stinging rebuff from the Queen led him to mount a case against Lopez, whose confession would be assured under interrogation: the Portuguese doctor would be 'cross-examined' until, one way or another, the 'truth' was forced out of him.

It seems the King of Spain had at some time in the past given Lopez a ruby ring. His accusers asked about it, but during the interrogation Lopez denied on oath it was of any significance. But another spy in custody told a different story, and Robert Cecil began to feel he had been a little hasty in his initial assessment—and, indeed, could have been wrong. That sealed Lopez's fate; he was doomed. Worn down by incessant questioning, he was shown the rack and he confessed to whatever the Earl of Essex and his henchmen cared to put before him. His guilt was dubious, but the Earl's violent personal grudge and desire to regain favour with the Queen carried the day.

A trial of sorts followed and Lopez, royal doctor or not, together with Ferreira and another conspirator, Tinoco, were sentenced to death as traitors.

The Queen hesitated to ratify the sentence. Such vacillation was her style, as famously seen in her delay in agreeing to the execution of her cousin, Mary Queen of Scots, in February 1587. It took almost four months of agonising indecision for her to eventually sanction the beheading.

In the doctor's case she also took four months—and, ever shrewd and used to an atmosphere of intrigue, she probably saw through the Earl of Essex and sensed an injustice had been perpetrated. However, she did eventually agree, and in June 1594 the men were dragged to Tyburn—where Marble Arch now stands, adjacent to London's Hyde Park—for their execution before a vast holiday crowd.

Lopez, our main interest, went to the gallows first. While standing on the scaffold he attempted to make a dying speech, doubtless to protest his innocence, but the excited and prejudiced crowd howled him down. Amid the uproar he was hurried to the gibbet and hanged, and—such was the law—was cut down while still alive, then castrated, disembowelled and quartered.

The last to hang was Tinoco. The job was botched: he was cut down too soon, more alive than dead, then struggled to his feet and took to his executioner and tried to strangle him. The crowd cheered at the feisty performance, but he was overpowered, held down and, without any further fuss about a re-hanging, was dispatched by the customary castration, disembowelment and gruesome quartering.

What cruel times they lived in.

To her credit, Elizabeth was merciful to the doctor's family—perhaps due to a twinge of conscience. It was usual to retain the property of a felon, but she allowed the widow to keep all her husband's goods and chattels, with one exception: she took possession of King Philip's ring. She slipped it onto her finger, where it stayed for the rest of her life.

John Frederick Struensee (1737–1772)

Another case—which makes the grumbles about government regulations by the doctors of today seem of little importance—concerns the rough justice dealt out by government officials in Denmark to Dr John Frederick Struensee, only 200 years ago.

In 1766, at the age of fifteen, Caroline Matilda, youngest sister of the British monarch, George III, and great aunt of the future Queen Victoria, was torn from her loving mother's arms and hurried away from the English court to marry her dissolute, decadent and debilitated first cousin, Christian VII, King of Denmark. It was a marriage arranged for political expediency, but even the English court's powerbrokers would have bridled at the match had they realised the Danish swain was a dedicated habitué of prostitutes, was syphilitic, and already had cerebral changes from the tertiary and final phase of this loathsome sexually transmitted disease.

In stark contrast, his young new wife, now called Queen Matilda, had been raised in a secluded, genteel and domesticated way as befitted a junior member of eighteenth-century British royalty, and was largely ignorant of the ways of the world. (Her father, Frederick, Prince of Wales, died before he could assume the throne, following, it is alleged, a blow on the head with a cricket ball.)

On the death of his mother, Christian's father had remarried and sired a second son, Ferdinand. On the old King's death, Christian's stepmother and now Dowager Queen, Juliana Maria, had dedicated herself to getting the young Ferdinand onto the throne. Despite all the court intrigue, the elder boy was rightly and legally regarded as the heir, so Christian was not only duly crowned, but married the sturdily built Matilda, who fell pregnant shortly after.

At the time the King's sexually transmitted diseases were being treated—albeit ineffectively, as there was then no cure—by Dr John Frederick

Struensee, and it was he who also attended Queen Matilda and the couple's new son. Struensee himself was the son of a clergyman, and though considered by some to be a 'libertine and free-thinker', was also regarded as a good doctor who tried in vain to dissuade the monarch from his licentious ways. It was a vain hope. Any change of behaviour was all too late anyway—and, as night follows day, his gentle if willing wife caught the contagious disease.

Besides attending the sick at court, Struensee had another ambition: he secretly coveted authority, command and, above all, power. He ruthlessly pursued these ends and by early 1771 had wormed his way up the political ladder to become prime minister of the country, as well as royal physician.

Some regard power as the greatest of all aphrodisiacs, and as the King slipped further and further into confused imbecility, the scandalously obvious flirtation that had developed between the royal physician and the Queen became more indiscreet than medical etiquette generally allows. Without putting too fine a point on it, and despite the transmittable malady from which the doctor knew his heart's desire suffered, they became lovers. At the same time, the certifiable monarch was conveniently confined to his apartments, out of the way—on the orders of the very same man who had supplanted Christian in his wife's bed.

Although she was by now a buxom nineteen-year-old in a loveless relationship, and Struensee was a personable, tall, flaxen-haired 33-year-old, intimacy between a Queen and her physician-cum-prime-minister was wildly, albeit excitingly, indiscreet. The scandal soon became an open secret and its shamelessness compounded when, after she was criticised for displaying more of her ample bosom than was thought appropriate, Prime Minister Struensee dismissed the prurient officials responsible for the observations with un-Danish expediency.

With that, the court powerbrokers agreed that enough was enough: Struensee had to go, and sooner rather than later. The Queen Dowager needed no second bidding to lend her support, as she had been looking for some time for an excuse to enter the succession fray. While the officials may have wanted to restore the old order, she was more devious and saw it as a back door to the throne for Ferdinand.

Things came to a head in late 1771. With the help of a pliant nobleman, the Dowager Queen bullied her stepson, the by-now witless and rambling King, into signing an instrument of arrest for the wanton pair.

Plans were laid for the deed to be done on 16 January 1772, at a psychologically unguarded moment for the couple. To add to the drama and comic-opera scenario, it was to be enacted following a grand ball at the palace that evening.

All the top echelon were at the glittering affair, and Matilda and Struensee danced before their appalled gaze with unbecoming abandon. The depth of her *décolletage* or splendour of her *embonpoint* is unrecorded, but eventually, having danced most of the night away, the star-crossed lovers retired to her apartment in seeming ignorance of their impending doom. As the doctor left the arms of his royal lover and returned to his own quarters, guards apprehended him on the stairs. He was hurried away in a hackney carriage to a nearby dungeon. The Queen was escorted to the northern fortress of Cronenborg Castle, accompanied by dragoons whose swords were drawn to prevent a sudden, but highly unlikely, dash to safety.

In his dank prison Dr Struensee was chained to a wall in such a way that he could neither sit nor stand properly and was left starving to ponder his fate. Thumbscrews were used to extract a 'confession', and to add to his unenviable situation, the Queen had recently had a second child and Struensee was declared the father. In view of the royal husband's parlous medical state, there was almost certainly some truth in this paternity claim.

The English court was outraged at the course of events involving one of their own, and George III wondered about declaring war, or at least sending his fleet into the Baltic. In the end he settled on dispatching his envoy to Denmark to vouchsafe a diplomatic solution ensuring Matilda's safety. Perhaps rather surprisingly, this was accomplished: the outcome was that the royal couple were divorced, the two children were left with the King, and Matilda sailed for her homeland.

The wicked stepmother was now in command, but her rapacious grasping of power was not the outcome hoped for by the Danish court, and there were murmurings for the return of Matilda, the rightful queen. More diplomatic exchanges took place, and by dint of some cloak-and-dagger machinations Matilda was approached in England to return to Denmark. She eventually agreed.

The decision must have involved a very generous settlement, for the tremendous risk she ran was surely obvious to all. And so it proved to be. Although apparently in perfect health on leaving England, within seven weeks of her return, Matilda, aged only 21, was dead. It was claimed she died from 'a contagious fever' caught from one of her domestics. So, after a short but turbulent and unfulfilled life, Matilda, Queen of Denmark and of Norway, was laid to rest in the town of Zell, not far from where she died.

Matilda's death occurred with questionable rapidity. Given that 'contagious fever' is a rather woolly and all-embracing diagnosis, and knowing the feelings of the wicked stepmother, it would be very surprising if some skulduggery was not involved. We shall never know.

But what of our main interest, the luckless Dr Struensee?

Having been tortured over several months and found guilty of treason for seducing the monarch's wife, on 28 April 1772 he was brought to the scaffold in chains. First he was forced to watch his servant being beheaded; such a quick death, however, was thought too good for the by-now terrified physician, for it was vengeance that was sought. So he was first doused with his servant's spilled blood—then he had his right hand chopped off. After a pause to allow the full horror to sink in, he was then disembowelled and finally quartered.

Struensee's head was fixed on a post, and his hacked-off right hand nailed below it. The four quarters of the body were dragged to a refuse dump outside the city and there placed in the centre of a horizontally fixed wagon wheel; the entrails were buried beneath its supporting staves. The remains were then left to be devoured by scavenging dogs and predatory birds.

The murder of an over-ambitious royal doctor was now complete, and no doubt the crowd went home feeling well satisfied at the outcome. And all this happened only 200-odd years ago.

3

Doctors to Charles I and Charles II

Charles I of England (1600–1649)

Born in Dunfermline, Scotland, in 1600, where his father reigned as James VI (later to become James I of England), as a young boy Charles was a sickly child, unable to speak until his fifth year—and, it is said, so weak in the ankles that to get about he had to crawl on his hands and knees until he was seven. Charles outgrew these very unusual disabilities, but was left with a stammer and became something of a scholar. In adulthood, Charles was looked after by one doctor, who by great good fortune was one of England's greatest ever, William Harvey. Their relationship became more than that of doctor and patient, for they became firm friends.

Dr William Harvey is best known for first describing the circulation of the blood around the body, a discovery he made in 1618, but the detail of which he did not publish until 1628. His finding was the one discovery, above all others, that allowed medicine to move out of the Dark Ages and open the way to medical practice as we know it today. Now in the British Museum, his book *Exercitatio Anatomica De Motu Cordis et Sanguinis in Animalibus* (The Anatomical Treatise on the Movement of the Heart and Blood in Animals), or *De Motu Cordis* for short, was written in the author's terrible handwriting in a mixture of Latin and English, held together by a lattice of lines, arrows and erasures and a number of errors. It is dedicated to his friend and patron, Charles I.

Born in 1578, William Harvey graduated with honours in Padua, Italy, in 1602, and returned to England in 1609, joining the staff of St Bartholomew's Hospital, London, where he was to work for 37 years. According to John Aubrey, the famous gossip of the times and author of *Brief Lives*, Harvey was a short, swarthy and testy man who invariably wore a dagger, which he was 'inclined to draw at the slightest provocation'.

In 1618, the year he discovered the circulation of the blood, he was appointed Physician-in-Extraordinary to King James I, whose son, Charles I, made him Physician-in-Ordinary on assuming the throne in 1625.

Charles took a great interest in Harvey's work and placed at his disposal the royal deer in Richmond Park for his experimental work. In 1640 Robert Hannah painted his famous picture of Harvey explaining to Charles and one of his sons, probably the younger Charles, the blood circulation in one of these deers. The picture now hangs in the Royal College of Physicians in Regents Park, London, dramatically positioned at the top of a sweeping staircase.

He brought out another book in 1651, which is regarded as the first publication by an English author on the art and craft of obstetrics.

Unfortunately, just when his expertise in obstetrics was needed, Harvey was not on hand on 11 May 1629 at Greenwich Palace to save the first-born child of Charles I.

The story goes that Queen Henrietta Maria, Charles' wife, had returned to Greenwich by barge from the city to begin her confinement, but fell as she was getting onto the landing stage. She went into labour two days later, six weeks premature. As this took place at an unplanned time, the local midwife had to be summoned—but she was so overcome on discovering the identity of the mother that she fainted away, leaving the Queen to cope as best she could without professional help. A royal prince and heir to the throne was delivered, immediately christened Charles. He promptly died.

It was feared that Henrietta would prove incapable of bearing another child, and that the Stuart dynasty was thus in jeopardy. But she did in fact have a healthy son almost exactly a year later, and to help overcome the memory of the earlier loss he was christened Charles too, and would later become Charles II of England.

Charles I and his great friend William Harvey became embroiled in the armed struggle, known as the English Civil War (1642–49), between supporters of the King (Cavaliers) and parliamentarians (Roundheads) led by Oliver Cromwell. It arose from constitutional, religious and economic differences between Charles and Members of his Parliament. All sections of society were affected and often families were divided by competing allegiances. Charles insisted on the 'divine right of kings' to rule; the elected Parliament disagreed. Starting with an indecisive engagement at Edgehill, the balance tipped towards the Roundheads, culminating in a crushing defeat of the Cavaliers at Naseby in 1645. Charles surrendered, escaped in 1646, was recaptured in 1648, and publicly beheaded on 30 January 1649.

In the meantime, back to William Harvey who, being a staunch Royalist, had his house in Whitehall, London, plundered by the rampaging Roundheads after their victory. Tragically, many of his papers and experimental results were lost to posterity.

Harvey, of course, could do little medically to help his king at his death on the scaffold. For Charles I, death was just a glint of steel and a shout from the crowd. There could be no prolonged deathbed scenes and multiple drug administrations that, as we shall see, accompanied his son's death. But he had been fortunate to have had such a great man attend his royal person during his pomp.

William Harvey died aged 79 in 1657, eight years after his royal patient and backer was executed. He is buried at Hempstead, a village near Cambridge; his grave is still there.

Charles II (1630–1685)

During the Civil War, in 1642, Charles I's son, later to become Charles II, had been forced into exile. After his father's execution he assumed the title of King while still on the Continent, but returned to Scotland in June that year and was proclaimed Charles II in Edinburgh. However, he had to wait until 1 January 1651 to actually be crowned, an event which took place at Scone. He invaded England not long afterwards, was defeated at Worcester and escaped to France, enduring many scrapes and near-misses of capture, to spend nine years in impoverished exile.

With the fall of Cromwell's Protectorate he returned in triumph to London on his birthday on 29 May 1660 and properly assumed his throne.

The Restoration court over which Charles II presided was a place of unceasing and brazen scandal. He—and it—revelled in the intrigue and sexual excesses which it spawned, and which in the end may have caused his death in 1685 at the comparatively early age of 55. He had numerous doctors, apothecaries and a druggist at his beck and call, and by happy chance for us three hundred years later, at his life's end he also had in attendance John Evelyn (1620–1706), one of England's great diarists, to record his—doubtless distressing—last few days.

Charles' principal doctor was Dr Charles Scarburgh (1616–1694). He was a graduate of Caius College, Cambridge, where he originally studied mathematics, but turned to medicine and graduated as an MD in 1646. He was a friend of the great William Harvey in Charles I's time, and became physician to Charles II in 1672. It was to Dr Scarburgh during his last days of prolonged agony that the Merry Monarch made his famous apology for being 'an unconscionable time a-dying'.

On that occasion Scarburgh had the aid—or more likely, hindrance—of eleven other medical personnel. With so many in attendance, each feeling compelled to have his say, capricious administration of polypharmacy would have been the inevitable result: a medical overkill, so to speak. This blunderbuss approach doubtless hastened Charles II's death, though the final outcome was probably never in doubt.

At Dr Scarburgh's elbow was Dr John Micklethwaite, President of the Royal College of Physicians, who because of his distinguished position was called in when Charles had his first apoplectic attack—violent convulsions—on 2 February 1685. Micklethwaite prescribed cinchona bark, an odd choice of treatment by our lights as it was used for malaria.

Also present was trainee apothecary Thomas Williams. In such company he was punching above his weight, but for reasons unknown he was an invitee. Williams bled the King, removing 16 ounces of blood (about 450 mL), gave him some black cherry julep, then removed 10 more ounces (say 300 mL) of blood. The therapeutic value of all this was dubious, as was the application of a 'Mrs Corbett's plaster' he slapped on somewhere on the body of the long-suffering king.

Even more doubtful was the attention sought of the royal barber, Ralph Foliard, who shaved the royal head on the supposition that it removed any weight pressing on the brain. The King's misery must have been compounded when, after this complete tonsure, cantharides—popularly known as Spanish fly—was rubbed into the shining pate. Taken by mouth, Spanish fly is better known as an aphrodisiac that allegedly acts by inflaming the urethra—the urinary passageway from the bladder to the outside. If indeed this was in the doctor's mind, it was about the last thing the fast-fading monarch required.

So what was the lead-up to all this empirical polypharmacy, as faithfully recorded by Evelyn?

The Merry Monarch was never short of female company and boasted several mistresses over the years. These included Frances Stuart, the Duchess of Richmond, whose likeness for centuries appeared on the reverse of some British coins, purporting to be Britannia. It showed her as a helmeted figure on a throne, trident in one hand and a large shield in the other. She modelled the pose in 1665.

There was the ex-orange seller from the Drury Lane theatre, Nell Gwynne, claiming to be 'the Protestant whore' when she once shouted at a crowd jeering about Charles' hated Catholic connections; the Duchess of Portsmouth, a favourite, and several others. It is said that from the various ladies he produced fifteen illegitimate children. He had a legal wife as well, Catherine of Braganza, but the union was childless—a state of affairs which, in view of his track record, caused some surprise in the court.

On the evening of 1 February 1685, Charles was holding court at Whitehall. The scene has been set by Evelyn, who wrote:

I can never forget the inexpressible luxury and profaneness, gaming and dissoluteness, and, as it were, total forgetfulness of God, (it being Sunday evening) which the day and night I was witness of. The King sitting and toying with his concubines, Portsmouth, Cleveland and Mazarine; a French boy singing love songs, whilst about 20 courtiers and other dissolute persons were at Basset around a large table, a bank of at least 2000 golden guineas before them. Six days later all was dust.

On Monday morning his attendants noticed their chief was unusually pale and that his speech was indistinct. Whilst being shaved, the King fell backwards with a cry and into the arms of Lord Ailesbury. He had violent convulsions, described as an apoplectic fit. The royal ablutions were always a time for hangers-on to mill about, and, by chance, the keeper of the 'royal crucible and retorts' (mixing bowls to catch blood, and glass jars) was on hand. Ever attentive, he whipped out the lancet, without which no self-respecting crucible-keeper should travel, and withdrew 16 ounces of blood (about 450 mL). This apparently gave immediate relief and allowed messengers to ride off rapidly in all directions to seek the court physicians. (The King paid his doctors £100 a year and, as one prescription later given was signed by fourteen doctors, it must have been an expensive indulgence.)

Six arrived fairly quickly and they ordered cupping glasses to be applied to the shoulders forthwith, together with deep scarifications. This removed another 8 ounces of blood (225 mL). Cupping consists of applying a kind of inverted wineglass-shaped container that has been flamed to burn the oxygen, and thus evacuate the glass of air. The negative pressure thus created inside the glass allows the flesh to be drawn in, and if the skin is cut, blood to be sucked out. It has an honoured lineage stretching to the Stone Age and is still used in southern Europe today. Its therapeutic use, however, is questionable.

To free the stomach of all impurities a strong ammoniacal emetic was given to induce vomiting, but as the King could only swallow part of this he was given a chaser of zinc sulphate in peony water. Strong purgation was then given, and to make doubly sure a succession of enemas—or clysters as they were then called—were administered. These comprised herbs, linseed oil, antimony wine and rock salt, and their rectal introduction anticipated an administrative principle which was evident in some maternity hospitals when I was a medical student 50 years ago—namely, their intromission should be 'high, hot and a hell of a lot'.

More fits were forthcoming, so a red-hot cautery was sent for and applied somewhere to the body. At all events there was a dramatic improvement. Within two hours consciousness was completely restored, and for the first time the King was able to give an account of his symptoms.

Instead of leaving well alone, the assembled medical faculty thought an encore was needed to relieve the pressure of the 'humours' of the brain. They induced sneezing which, in the presence of looseness of the bowels, is a potentially explosive situation, but one that would at least divert His Majesty's attention from his apoplexy.

The doctors' ingenuity, being applied to a compliant patient, seemed to know no bounds. Noxious ointments of tar and pigeon dung were applied to the soles of the feet and a blistering plaster of cantharides was again administered. Soothing draughts of barley and liquorice were given to the monarch to treat the treatment; supper consisted of broth and ale made without hops. With this, therapeutic creativeness rested from its labours for the day.

By Tuesday twelve physicians had come to justify their stipend and found the patient much improved, a success which stimulated them into pursuing treatment along the same lines. More black cherry water was administered, and more blood taken—10 ounces (about 300 mL) this time 'just in case'. The principle behind letting of blood was that with its flow, so too was removed the 'badness' from within the body. Anyway, it was all in all a day of rest.

Wednesday again brought a confidence that only a pint of senna tea and the letting of 8 ounces of blood (225 mL) could enhance. A bulletin was issued by doctors stating that in a few days the King would be freed from his distemper, a pious hope fostered by ignorance. As the assembled doctors had impeccable backgrounds the pronouncement was taken as a kind of *ex cathedra* statement, and so some low-key celebrations were thought to be in order by all concerned.

They had spoken and imbibed too soon. Scarcely had the ink dried on the optimistic bulletins and the back-slapping stopped when Charles had a series of fresh convulsions. The skull of some recently executed malefactor was produced, flamed, and spirit of burnt skull at once administered, a trump card the playing of which was contemporaneously regarded as a sure harbinger of impending doom. It was said to excite horror in the patient and so act by suggestion to scare away the evil spirits. I am sure the King hoped it would do the same to his doctors. It was not to be.

By Thursday the King's ministers began to get restive, not unreasonably wanting to know the diagnosis—a piece of intelligence the doctors would have loved themselves. Not only were they running out of ideas, but there were not too many areas of the royal body that had not already been assaulted by lancets, scarifiers, bleeding cups, blisterers or unctions.

Someone thought of intermittent fever, or malaria as we now call it. Unknown in England now, in the seventeenth century it was endemic in the low-lying fen district of eastern England. Indeed, Oliver Cromwell himself, who came from those parts, had been a sufferer, but the treatment of the day—cinchona bark—was so bitter that even that hard-boiled old Roundhead could not force it down. Never mind, try anything, so Charles II had it at three-hourly intervals. That was the prescription signed by all fourteen of his physicians, and it was on that very day that the dying King made his famous utterance about taking an unconscionable time a-dying. It sounds more like a prayer for deliverance than a real apology.

It was also on that day that he asked his brother to bring a priest. The only one available was John Huddleston, a Benedictine monk. Because he was a

Catholic—a faith unacceptable to the establishment since the dissolution of the monasteries by Henry VIII 150 years previously—Huddleston dressed in wig and gown and, thus disguised, pronounced absolution and administered extreme unction. So the Merry Monarch, having lived as a token Protestant, died a Catholic. (By a quirk of fate his brother and successor, James II, was an openly committed Catholic, and on account of it lost the throne three years later.)

At dawn the next day, Friday 6 February, there was an understandable air of gloom in the medical camp, although the King's mind remained clear. Suddenly, however, the monarch had an attack of breathlessness, so was bled yet again whilst his doctors regrouped. Desperate times need desperate measures, so he was given 'Raleigh's Stronger Antidote', an extract of an enormous number of herbs, Goa Stone*, powdered oyster shells and Oriental bezoar stone. A bezoar stone was very difficult to lay hands on because it was a concretion formed in the stomach of an East Indian goat and was believed to have mystical properties in destroying poisons and reanimating vital powers.

That finally did it, for by 8.30 that morning the King's speech began to fail, by ten o'clock he was comatosed and at noon he died, released from the nocuous, though well meant, ministrations of the royal doctors.

---

* A Goa Stone is a paste of exotic tropical ingredients, e.g. amethyst, rubies and coral, and made in the Portuguese colony of Goa in India. Unlike a bezoar stone, it is man-made.

The following day a post-mortem was carried out and the King was found to have dilatation of the blood vessels on the surface of the brain. His heart was enlarged and there were adhesions in the chest from a previous attack of pleurisy.

There were rumours that Charles II had been poisoned but, with the various inconclusive tests then available, no evidence was found. If in fact he had been poisoned it was surely by the overzealous doctors in attendance. He may have had a form of inflammation of the kidneys or nephritis (later called Bright's disease after the man who first described it in the mid-nineteenth century), but it seems the renal system appeared to be largely normal.

Probably the most likely cause of death was raised blood pressure, either as an entity of itself or following microscopic damage to the kidneys caused by gout, possibly from an attack of that form of arthritis as being recorded shortly before he died. At this distance in time it is difficult to make a firm diagnosis.

Charles II had ruled over a court that was a byword in sexual excesses, gambling and riotous living generally. He himself revelled in the intrigue and sexual jousts which it spawned. In the main he had little contact with the realities of day-to-day life in England, although he gained general approbation for his consideration and leadership during the Great Fire of London.

In the end he suffered patiently and with regal fortitude the degrading ministrations of his incompetent and bewildered physicians—all fourteen of them. A commoner would probably have been allowed to die with dignity, attended by a single doctor working without being bombarded with expressions of differing opinions, each more outrageous than its predecessor. But the King's exalted position led to a frantic search for an instant miracle: 58 drugs were administered in a five-day period, and from time to time his attendants had to force open his mouth and he frequently vomited them back up. The efforts of his physicians and surgeons were applauded at the time as being courageous and exhaustive. That is certainly true, but their predictable failure made his death pitiful and painful. Really, it was being a king that killed him.

Several years before the Merry Monarch's death, his friend John Wilmot, Earl of Rochester—like Charles II a womanising reprobate—wrote for his sovereign lord a rather scurrilous epitaph. It went:

> Here lies a great and mighty king
> Whose promise none relies on;
> He never said a foolish thing,
> Nor ever did a wise one.

As Rochester died five years before his King, the epitaph was never chiselled on stone. Instead came the witty rejoinder from Charles II, typifying the laid-back nature of his court and the man himself: 'This is very true: for my words are my own, and my actions are my ministers.'

4
The incompetent doctors of Mad George III

The British king George III (1738–1820) was a Hanoverian who followed his grandfather, George II, onto the English throne in 1760. He was aged 21 at the time and, nominally at least, was to be monarch for an incredible 60 years. The reason the monarchy skipped a generation was that his father, Frederick, Prince of Wales, met an untimely end following a blow from a cricket ball. He did not die right there at the wicket in mid-match, but some months later as a result of an abscess that developed beneath the site of the blow. It was a most unusual way to 'get out', so to speak.

In his youth George III was said to have been indolent, indecisive, timid, slow-witted and highly sexed. His conversation was punctuated by meaningless questions such as, 'What? What?' or 'Hey? Hey?' Though this invited ridicule and parody, his subjects regarded him as a kindly and honest—if somewhat eccentric—man. As he competently ran a farm in the grounds of Windsor Castle, a little later in life he became affectionately known as Farmer George.

But he is most famous in history for the state of his mind, which over quite a few years displayed a steady disassociation with reality. In 1762 at the age of 24 he had his first recorded delusional episode when he seized the lower branch of an oak tree, shook it and engaged it in conversation, supposing it to be the King of Prussia. His doctor 'bled' him several times and he was 'blistered'. After about two months the symptom passed, but there were several lesser hushed-up episodes over the next few years. It was not until 1788, when George was 50, that a more sinister happening took place—one that was to rock the British establishment.

In June that year he began to suffer severe abdominal pains, and a month later he became excitable and voluble, said at the time to have been brought on by his failure to change out of wet stockings. His excitability subsided, but returned in October, together with constipation, sweating, insomnia, agitation, confusion and, eventually, fits. As it was reported at the time, any medicines given seemed 'not to have repelled the fever upon the brain'.

His doctor, or apothecary as he was called then, was Sir George Baker, President of the Royal College of Physicians and a fine practitioner where ordinary illnesses were concerned. Son of a vicar in Devonshire, he received his MD in 1756, and after practising in his home county moved to London in 1761, where he soon acquired a large following, especially among the aristocracy, and eventually an appointment to the royal household.

Besides being the monarch's doctor, Baker had two other claims to fame: he was the dedicatee of Thomas Gray's well-known poem, 'Elegy Written in a Country Churchyard', and in 1767 wrote a paper that made him even more famous than being the King's doctor. It was entitled *Inquiry Concerning the*

Cause of Epidemic Colic of Devonshire. Briefly, he proved that the common colicky abdominal pains which occurred in that part of England's south-west, and very rarely elsewhere, was caused not by over-indulgence in the renowned local alcoholic beverage, cider, but by the lead it contained. The lead had leached into the liquid from the lead-lined cider presses used by the apple farmers of Devon to make their cider.

As a result of his discovery Baker was attacked by his neighbours, denounced from the pulpit as a faithless son of Devon who was putting the area's principal industry in jeopardy—and anyway, living as he did in London, what did he know? His detractors claimed the griping stomach pains were from the 'bad humours' of the body. They did, however, finally remove the lead lining from the apple presses and Devonshire colic disappeared, never to return.

But back to the madness of George III, who was being looked after by a physician who was very competent, but failing in his treatment of the King's mental state. Baker put it down to gout brought on by a diet of sauerkraut and lemonade (not cider, you will note). He dispatched the patient to Cheltenham Spa to take the waters and to use rhubarb pills as a purge.

Initially there was some lessening of the symptoms, but by October they were back, supplemented by the added nuisance of skin rashes and manic behaviour. The King talked incessantly and the Queen commented that his eyes had become so deep and so dark they were 'like blackcurrant jelly'.

As the condition became more florid poor Dr Baker, sensing dismissal was

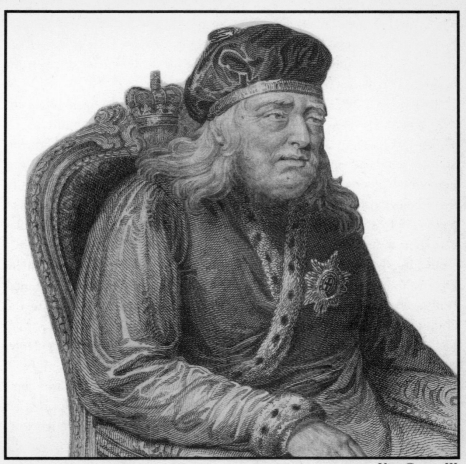

King George III

in the wind, declared himself sick and left the scene voluntarily. He was succeeded by Dr Richard Warren, a society doctor who reputedly examined his own tongue each morning in the mirror and paid himself for doing so by transferring a guinea from one pocket to another.

By January 1789, Dr Warren considered the King too deranged to govern the country. This was serious stuff, so an authority on mental conditions, Dr Thomas Monro from Bethlem Hospital—better known as Bedlam, the London hospital where advanced mentally deranged people were incarcerated—was summoned. His brutal methods had already attracted the disapprobation of the theologian John Wesley, and in a rare lucid moment George refused to be treated by someone from that institution, so Monro was dismissed after a very short tenure.

Eventually the Prime Minister and supporter of the royal family, William Pitt the Younger, stepped in and entrusted the King to the care of Dr Francis Willis, who had made his mark on medical history by putting forward the notion that insanity was curable.

Francis Willis (1718–1807) had not started out as a doctor but a clergyman, having taken holy orders before gaining an MD at Oxford in 1759. Because of his double qualification in theology and medicine, he was commonly known as 'Dr Duplicate'. In 1769 he was appointed a physician at an asylum in Lincoln, rather insensitively called 'the House for Wrongheads', where he successfully treated several cases of mental disorder.

His favoured form of treatment was to deploy a mixture of psychological bullying, morale-boosting, and fixing the eye to obtain dominance, all supplemented by blistering. A very proactive practitioner, Willis also insisted on restraint (usually with a straitjacket) and a mixture of emetics, purges, bleeding, long walks, the application of leeches and, for uplifting the morale, being dressed neatly. Willis had come accompanied by his son, Dr John Willis, and three burly keepers with straitjackets and a chair in which the patient could be strapped down and beaten if thought necessary. When appointed to the royal household he met with considerable opposition, but maintained that the King would recover, especially if moved to Kew Palace where long walks could be taken more easily.

In view of the King's parlous state, the prudent House of Commons passed a Bill of Regency that allowed his replacement if things persisted. Before the Bill was promulgated, however, George improved dramatically under the Willis regime, and on 26 February 1789 a 'cessation of illness' was announced. It was almost certainly due to a natural remission in the malady; it was to be twelve years before another attack occurred.

With the King more or less back to his old self, a Thanksgiving service was held at St Paul's Cathedral on 23 April, St George's Day. The father-and-son physicians took credit for the cure, not realising it was simply a natural progression of the disease. Their reward was £1000 a year for 21 years for Dr Francis, and £650 a year for the rest of his life for Dr John.

A number of contemporary diagnoses were made: consequential madness, fatuity, nervous fever—and, a century later, manic depressive psychosis. It was felt at the time that George III was taking his job as King too seriously, but we now know the true cause was almost certainly something quite different, namely an inborn error of metabolism.

During his life George had five further attacks, with a similar cluster of symptoms, as well as lameness, paraesthesia (numbness), photophobia, insomnia lasting several days, disorientation, hallucinations and disinhibited behaviour. Each attack lasted about two months, except the last, which persisted for ten years and was complicated by total deafness and blindness from cataracts. He must have presented as a tragic figure and it was during this period that his son, also called George, took over as Regent. The era became known as The Regency.

Treatment remained brutal, but though undignified, barbaric and degrading as it may have been, the monarch lived to be 82 and, including The Regency while he was still nominally King, he ruled for 60 years, the second-longest reign in British history after Queen Victoria's 64 years.

The repetitive triad of abdominal pain, neuritis and mental disturbance is the hallmark of an inherited metabolic disorder called acute intermittent porphyria. But not until 1966 was it mooted by the mother-and-son research team Ida MacAlpine and Richard Hunter that this may have been the genesis of George III's illness.

George had fifteen children (he himself was one of nine) and as porphyria is transmitted genetically, it should not have been difficult to find other cases in the family. Indeed, this is how MacAlpine and Hunter came onto it when they were writing a history of psychiatry, and as James I had written a book on witchcraft, they were looking carefully at him.

A feature of the malady is that when particular metabolites become excessive in the blood, the skin becomes sensitive to sunlight, and James, they found, suffered from a very delicate skin.

Another manifestation is the excretion of dark-red pigmented porphyrins in the urine, which appears bluish-red if it is stood for some time. It seems that James I occasionally passed urine so red he himself described it as being like 'Alicante wine'. He also had attacks of colic and depression. Renal stones, or calculi, were ruled out as a cause of the urine discolouration as James' kidneys were found to be normal at post-mortem.

Furthermore, his mother, Mary Queen of Scots, suffered frequently from abdominal and leg pains, paraesthesia and melancholia. When beheaded she was found to be bald beneath a wig; perhaps a manifestation of the skin condition.

George III was descended from these Stuarts, and when his medical history was carefully reviewed in 1966, surprise, surprise, there was found four recorded episodes of blue-red urine being passed over a 40-year period.

When the King died, his son the Prince Regent, now George IV, was too ill to attend the funeral on account of abdominal pains. The status of his urine is not known.

George IV's only child, Charlotte, died after a delivery lasting 55 hours. The child was stillborn. It was a sequence of events not untypical in acute overwhelming porphyria. Knowing nothing of this, her unfortunate obstetrician, Sir Richard Croft, committed suicide thinking his neglect had killed the heir to the throne.

George IV's brother, William IV, seems to have been clear, as was the child of a younger brother, Edward, the father of Queen Victoria.

So King George III was not mad, or at least if he was mentally disturbed it was due to an organic and nowadays treatable cause. So for 58 years George suffered grievously from his affliction, pitifully from its treatment, and miserably from its management by a battery of royal doctors who were using an armoury of therapies, the worth of which they were ignorant, while trying to care for a condition of which they knew nothing.

But perhaps he did marginally better than his counterpart over the Channel, Louis XVI, who, within four years of George's spontaneous recovery in February 1789, lost his head and crown in one fell swoop of the guillotine.

5
Death of a prince and princess

On the night of 18 February 1818, at about two o'clock in the morning, Sir Richard Croft, accoucheur to the British royal household and one of the 'super surgical specialists' on call to the royal presence, shot himself dead.

The genesis of this tragedy started on 3 November 1817 when Princess Charlotte, the only child of George, the Prince Regent and heir to the British throne, went into labour with her first child. All knew that one day it was highly likely the infant would become the British monarch, a scenario that must have lain heavily on Croft, her obstetrician.

Richard Croft was born in 1762 and as a young man took the usual method of entry into the medical profession at the time by becoming an apprentice to an apothecary. This apothecary was a Mr Chawner, who worked in the small picturesque town of Tutbury near the border of Staffordshire and Derbyshire in the English Midlands; it was in Tutbury Castle that Mary Queen of Scots had been imprisoned two centuries earlier. Having done his stint with the apothecary, Croft then progressed to St Bartholomew's Hospital in London to walk the wards as a senior medical student.

After graduating he returned to Tutbury and became a partner of Chawner. His first big medical moment came in 1790 when, aged 28, he attended the third confinement of the famed—perhaps infamous—courtesan Georgiana, wife of the fifth Duke of Devonshire. She divided her time between Chatswood House in Derbyshire, which was fairly near to Tutbury, and London, but as she neared her due date with this pregnancy she was in Paris. Croft's father-in-law, Dr Thomas Denman, had delivered the Duchess's previous two daughters, but felt too old to make the arduous journey from London to France. Croft was said to be a gifted and ambitious obstetrician who was sensitive to his patient's needs—or perhaps in Georgiana's case, whims—and robust enough to withstand the rigours of Continental travel. It was a long way to travel for a birth, and Croft arrived just in the nick of time to deliver a longed-for boy, the Marquess of Hartington.

When his father-in-law, Dr Denman, died in 1815, Croft inherited his London practice and left Tutbury and country practice forever. The new position boasted a large obstetrical following, including many members of the aristocracy, and it was eighteen months later that he was asked to look after Princess Charlotte during her first pregnancy. His experience and charm seem to have attracted the invitation, and at the age of 53 he must have seen plenty of obstetrical problems in his time.

Croft has been described as a diffident and sensitive man who was given to anxiety, even though he had a conservative attitude to managing childbirth: there were no heroics or chancy decisions in his work. He made no contributions to the medical literature of the day and was essentially a 'hands-on' man, whose integrity was held in high standing within the profession.

And now some background about Charlotte. Charlotte's grandfather happened to be the incumbent monarch, George III, who by 1817 was so mentally disturbed as to be out of contact with reality. In recent years it has been thought that his 'madness' was due to porphyria, one of a group of rare inherited disorders arising from an inborn error of metabolism. Prominent features of the condition include a bluish discolouration developing in the urine if it is left standing for a short period of time, sensitivity of the skin to sunlight, abdominal pains, and most obviously mental disturbances. In female sufferers it can also cause miscarriage.

George III and his wife, Queen Charlotte, had fifteen children, almost all of whom produced broods of bastard children, who, because of their illegitimacy, could have no claim to the throne. Because his eldest son, George, was properly married to Princess Caroline of Brunswick, their daughter, Charlotte, was legitimate, and so held a unique place in the order of succession.

Yet even Charlotte's birth had been surrounded by controversy. In 1782, at the age of twenty, her father George entered a morganatic marriage with a Mrs Fitzherbert. Not only was she a Roman Catholic, but her inamorato had married without the King's consent, making the union invalid under the Royal Marriage Act of 1722.

And so, in 1795, the Prince Regent cast about for an acceptable wife. He chose a gauche, unattractive and apparently rather malodorous princess, Caroline of Brunswick. It is said that on the wedding night George was so drunk and appalled at his bride's unattractiveness that he slept on the hearth rug. However, he was sober enough in the morning to consummate the marriage. Though said to have been their only act of intercourse during the whole of their lives together, by the greatest good fortune, from the dynastic viewpoint, it was sufficient: Caroline became pregnant.

Charlotte was born in January 1796 and the royal couple immediately separated, although Caroline did make a vain attempt to attend her lawful husband's eventual coronation in 1820.

As a child Charlotte suffered recurrent attacks of abdominal pain and alternating excitement and depression, which has led to the view that she too suffered from porphyria, though the character of her urine is unknown. Nonetheless, she grew into an attractive, though rather lonely, young lady.

In May 1816 she married Prince Leopold of Saxe-Coburg in what seems to have been a love match. After one miscarriage she fell pregnant again early in 1817, and on 1 October Mrs Griffiths, the attendant midwife-cum-wet nurse, took up residence in the royal house at Claremont.

A week later Dr Croft also moved in and waited for labour to begin. By this time the Princess was so large that twins were suspected.

Dr Croft occupied Leopold's dressing-room, next to Charlotte's bedroom, and in attendance as protocol decreed were eleven officers of state, including the Archbishop of Canterbury, the Bishop of London, the Lord Chancellor and—enigmatically—the Secretary of State for War, together with several ladies of the court. The gentlemen sat discreetly in an ante-chamber.

Charlotte finally went into labour at 7 a.m. on Monday 3 November, about two weeks overdue.

Labour proceeded slowly, very slowly. At 11 a.m. on Tuesday Croft rolled back his cuffs and performed a vaginal examination. Minimal dilation was noted and contractions were irregular. A second more senior obstetrician was called, Dr John Simms, as well as the royal physician. Though a senior man at 69, Simms was more interested in botany than childbirth: he had established the renowned herbarium at Kew. As he was not known to the Princess, Simms stayed in the next room while Crofts relayed his finding through the open door. Nothing could be more conducive to causing misunderstanding and confusion in the hurly-burly of the delivery room.

By 9 p.m. on Tuesday, after 36 hours in labour, the neck of Charlotte's womb (cervix) was fully dilated, but she was too weak to push. Croft dithered and Simms advised a hands-off approach. Croft had brought obstetrical forceps but refrained from using them, although with a full dilation it would have been the ideal moment to apply them. Perhaps the baby's head was not in the correct position, but this detail was not recorded.

At noon on Wednesday 5 November, dark green meconium was in evidence. This is the baby's bowel discharge and an ominous sign of foetal distress. That, night after 55 hours in labour, Charlotte delivered by her own efforts a stillborn boy, weighing 9 lb (about 4 kg). Dr Simms came in again and tried to resuscitate the baby, without success. Charlotte had a retained placenta, so while heroics on the baby were being performed, Croft did a difficult manual removal of this afterbirth.

Charlotte must have been completely exhausted by her labours, especially as during the night she began to haemorrhage, became excited and breathless, and had a thread-like pulse. She may have had a pulmonary clot; or the excitation and dyspnoea may have been a manifestation of acute porphyria. Later she became disorientated and irritable. Whatever the exact cause, at 2 a.m. on Thursday 6 November 1817, the heir to the British throne died.

A post-mortem was performed by George III's Physician-in-Ordinary. Blood was found in various cavities including the sac surrounding her heart, the pericardium. The doctor's report stated the cause of death was obscure, but today we know that her life may have been saved by the early use of forceps, and/or a more careful placental removal, resulting in less blood loss. A statue still stands today in St George's Chapel, Windsor Castle, depicting Princess Charlotte and her dead son ascending to heaven.

Sensitive and introspective, Croft, the royal obstetrician, must have brooded on what could or should have been done, for he knew as well as anyone that the stillborn child, had he lived, would one day have become King of England. He surely blamed himself too much, for Charlotte's delivery was always going to be difficult. She was a lady having her first child, the baby was large and suffering delay, and anaesthetics were not to be invented for another 30 years, so regrettably caesarean section was not an option.

The day after the tragedy, Croft wrote to Baron Stockmar, the personal physician of the child's father, saying, 'My mind is in a pitiable state. God grant that you yourself, or anyone dear to you, should ever suffer what I have experienced at this moment.'

Dr Croft continued to work until 18 February 1818, three months after the deaths, when he attended the labour of the wife of the royal chaplain in Wimpole Street, London. He retired to bed at 11 p.m. to await developments; at 2 a.m. the chaplain heard a noise, like the falling of a chair. An hour later the cleric went to wake the doctor and found him in bed with a discharged pistol in each hand and the muzzles pressed on the side of his head.

Croft was buried in St James Church, Piccadilly, beneath a simple marble plaque.

Charlotte's father later became George IV. When he died, the crown went first to George III's third son, William. He had ten illegitimate children, who could not claim the throne, and two legitimate children, who had died in infancy. On William's demise in 1837, the crown went to the eighteen-year-old daughter of George III's fourth son, Edward.

She became Queen Victoria.

6
Queen Victoria's doctors

A demanding patient and a chronic complainer, Queen Victoria (1819–1901) had a posse of doctors to look after her health. She employed a live-in Resident Medical Attendant as her personal general practitioner and to attend to her family and below-stairs staff. He was not, however, a member of the official household, which meant he could have breakfast and lunch with the ladies- and gentlemen-in-waiting, but was not permitted to dine at the royal table unless invited by the Queen herself. He had to accompany her when she moved from palace to palace: from Buckingham Palace in central London to Osborne House on the Isle of Wight (her favourite), Windsor Castle, Balmoral Castle in Scotland and so on. Further, she commonly holidayed in the south of France and visited her close relatives in Germany, so the doctor led a peripatetic life, with little time for himself and hardly any home life at all. For all this excoriating disruption, his salary was a parsimonious £400 (about £28,000 today) a year—but at least he lived and ate in elegant surroundings.

From the medical point of view, however, he was not alone: there was also at the regal beck and call a large medical back-up team, in a hierarchical system that survives to this day. The top consultants were the Physicians-in-Ordinary and Surgeons-in-Ordinary. The senior physician was called Head of the Medical Department and the senior surgeon, Sergeant-Surgeon. This latter's appellation did not indicate any army connection: 'sergeant' is derived from the Latin verb *servio*, meaning to serve or wait on. The first recorded Sergeant-Surgeon was William Hobbes in 1461 when Edward IV came to the throne. Then came a break in the records, but since 1530, when Henry VIII's famous surgeon Thomas Vicary held the position, the line has been unbroken to this day.

Under these chief medical men (always men) were lesser medical lights. Numbers in each category varied, but generally there were three Physicians and three Surgeons-Extraordinary on call to attend to not only Queen Victoria herself, but her large household as well. When not needed they carried on with their lucrative private practice. In the nineteenth-century court they were paid £200 a year for what was essentially a part-time job.

These Surgeons-Extraordinary were well-regarded medical men on probation, as it were, and if they behaved themselves and proved to be competent, many, but not all, would eventually be promoted to 'Ordinary' status. The complete medical staff comprised only men, for the simple reason that at that time there were no qualified female doctors in existence. Led by Elizabeth Garrett Anderson, women did not begin to appear on the medical scene until late in Victoria's reign, but none ever got the regal nod.

There were also 'super specialists' on call such as obstetricians, oculists, ear, nose and throat surgeons, and so on. There were no psychiatrists. At a lower level were the apothecaries, usually younger men. Their role was not easily defined, but they were like back-up general practitioners and were divided into two classes: apothecaries to the household who attended the staff but not the royal family; and apothecaries to 'the Person', who acted as general practitioners to the royal personage and members of her family if needed. They never became top doctors. All these medical acolytes helped prevent the nervous Queen Victoria from descending into a dither of anxiety, especially in her latter years.

So who were some of the more famous of these medical knights of the Victorian era, and what was the demanding task they had to perform?

The first well-known medico was Dr (later Sir) James Clark, who appeared early on in Victoria's reign and was prominent at the death of her consort, Prince Albert, which was perhaps the one event that caused most trauma in the Queen's life. So let's look at the passing of Albert, Prince Consort, and see where Clark fitted in.

Princess Diana died as a result of one of the great killers of the twentieth century: road trauma. Nearly 140 years previously, Albert died from one of the great killers of the nineteenth century: typhoid fever.

It was on the night of 14 December 1861 that Albert died at Windsor Castle. At the time the 'germ' theory of disease, which put forward bacteria as a cause of illness, had not yet been propounded: 'Acts of God' and the miasma

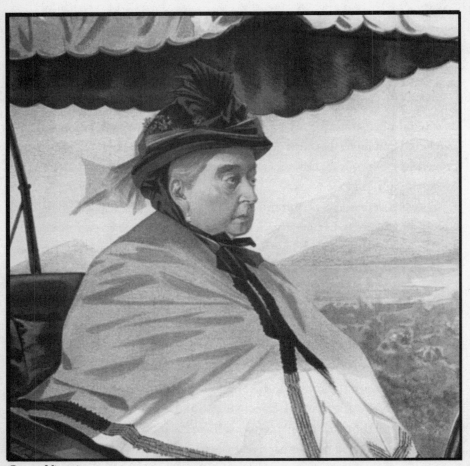

Queen Victoria

theory—in which bad smells and the like were the cause of illness—still held sway. It was not until the 1880s that French scientist Louis Pasteur connected the bacteria he saw down his microscope with a host of infectious diseases. As a result, in 1861 many irrelevant factors were being blamed for the death of the Prince. Besides miasma, one of the more unusual events—interpreted as a bad omen which was said to trigger his disease—was a sermon delivered at Crathie Church, Balmoral, at the end of the summer holiday two months previously. The minister had taken as his text, 'Prepare to meet thy God'. Later, in December, people remembered that sermon and put two and two together.

Blame was also laid on a change in palace doctors. Sir James Clark, the long-time incumbent, retired in 1860 and a Dr William Baly was appointed. Within months poor old Baly was killed in a railway accident—certainly an unusual way to go at that time, and once again seen as a highly portentous occurrence in the emotionally charged environment of the royal sick room.

The serious-minded Prince himself had an understandable fear of typhoid, so when he received news on 6 November 1861 that his German cousin, Prince Ferdinand, had died of the malady—an upset followed two days later by news of the same fate befalling two other cousins, Pedro V, King of Portugal, whom he 'had loved like a son', and Pedro's brother—he really had the breeze up.

The Queen herself had an even more novel theory as to the basis of Albert's fever. Their eldest son, Edward (later to become King Edward VII), was a student at Cambridge at the time and during the long summer vacation in 1861 had joined an army camp in the Curragh, Ireland. There he was introduced to a beautiful actress, Nellie Clifden. It seems the brazen and shameless hussy inveigled the heir to the throne into bed for his first sexual joust, where, it is rumoured she later said, 'he showed remarkable biological aptitude'.

The Clifden scandal eventually reached the ears of Edward's parents. They were mortified. Few, of course, were more Victorian in their outlook than the Queen herself. In high dudgeon Albert confronted and upbraided the now contrite Edward for his behaviour, and although they apparently smoothed things over, the Queen never really forgave her son and blamed him for the death of his father.

The Prince Consort's illness started on 22 November when he visited the British Army's Staff College at Sandhurst. He got soaking wet while reviewing the passing parade and developed a fever. Three days later, still feverish, he went to Cambridge to remonstrate with Edward over the Clifden affair. When Albert returned to Windsor Castle he complained of feeling at a 'very low ebb'.

He attended church on 29 November, but felt ill with nausea, weakness and loss of appetite. By 2 December his tongue was dry and brown, probably from dehydration—possibly kidney failure—and he became restless and depressed. Significantly, diarrhoea set in, whereupon the highly regarded but retired Dr Clark was summoned. Following the untimely death of Dr Baly, Clark had been reinstated as chief attending physician, and he now assured the Queen there was no cause for alarm; it was just a 'low fever'.

Let us leave the toxic and feverish Albert there on his bed of pain, with his wife crying helplessly (she later recorded in her diary that she felt as though her 'heart must break'), to ask: just who was this Sir James Clark?

A Scotsman, he was born in 1788, so was 73 when summoned to see Albert. As a school leaver he had intended to study law, and when still in his teens took the appropriate degree at Aberdeen University. However, Scotland at the time seems to have been the world's most fertile nursery of marine engineers and doctors, so he decided to go with the tide, electing to then pursue the less rigorous of these two popular disciplines by studying medicine at Edinburgh.

He graduated in 1809 and immediately entered the navy. Two of the ships on which he was serving were wrecked, but he survived to see out the Napoleonic Wars, at the conclusion of which he retired from the sea to start a medical practice in Rome. Over the next seven years he attended mainly the well-bred and well-heeled upper crust of the local English colony. One of his patients not in that genteel group was John Keats, the doctor-cum-poet who was coughing out his last tubercular years in the Eternal City and whom we shall meet later in the book.

During his holiday journeys in Europe, Clark visited the spa town of Carlsbad, Bohemia, where his interest in the local medicinal waters attracted the attention of another visitor, Prince Leopold, later to become King of the Belgians. It was a most propitious meeting, for when Clark returned to

England in 1826, Leopold appointed him his personal physician and he was able to set himself up as a high-society medical man. Medical fame also soon came to him when he published a well-researched article on the influence of climate on chest diseases. In 1834 Leopold recommended him as physician to the Duchess of Kent, mother of the future Queen Victoria. By natural progression, upon her succession to the throne in 1837, Clark was appointed Physician-in-Ordinary to the royal household.

Hence 24 years later it was he who was recalled from retirement to the bedside of Prince Albert in the early winter of 1861. Let us return there too.

On 6 December, two weeks after the onset of Albert's malaise, rose-coloured spots appeared on the royal torso. That did it—Clark now had no doubt about the diagnosis: typhoid. The Queen was told the worst; the official medical bulletin, however, spoke only of 'a feverish cold which was likely to continue for some time, but there were no unfavourable symptoms'.

By 10 December the Prince was weak, confused and rambling. The word 'typhoid' derives from the Greek *typhos*, meaning smoke or cloud, and refers to the floating confusion so typical of the late stages of the condition. More physicians were added to the entourage. Cyanosis, or a bluish tinge to the skin—especially the lips—then became apparent. It was an ominous sign of heart failure.

In the 1860s there were few trained nurses and only the indigent went to hospital, so Albert was looked after at home by servants and his daughters in the Blue Room at Windsor, the same room in which George IV and William IV had died before him. The Queen—or Weibchen, 'little wife', as her German husband Albert used to call her—had sprinkled his bedsheets with Eau de Cologne. While lying ethereally pale and breathless in bed, he was surrounded by all kinds of well-meaning hangers-on, from the Queen, their children, the Dean of Windsor, the tutor to the Prince of Wales, his private secretaries and a brace or two of generals; in all 20 people. The rather bizarre deathbed scene is shown in a colour lithograph in the possession of the Wellcome Institute for the History of Medicine trustees.

On the afternoon of 14 December a bulletin was issued to say the Prince was critical. Six hours later he was dead.

Queen Victoria and the *Times* newspaper praised the efforts of the doctors: others were not so sure. Lord Clarendon thought Dr Clark and his assistant Dr Holland were not average old women . . . they are 'not fit to attend a sick cat'.

In fact, by contemporary standards, with no knowledge of bacteria, they did their best given that the city's drinking water and adjacent sewerage system—home of the typhoid germ—was a public-health disaster zone. In 1861 untreated sewage flowed into the Thames, and untreated domestic drinking water was drawn from further down the river. There was no difficulty in acquiring typhoid; it mattered little whether you lived in a royal palace or a terraced slum.

Over the years there had been several well-recorded typhoid outbreaks. One was at Windsor Castle itself in 1859, when 30 royal servants were affected, three of whom died.

In October 1871, ten years after Albert's death from the disease, his son Prince Edward (of the Clifden affair) also contracted typhoid while staying at Londesborough Lodge in Yorkshire. Bulletins were issued by Sir William Jenner, Dr Gull and other doctors who were in attendance several times a day for the entire fortnight of the party. They were so gloomy in nature that the nation almost abandoned hope. A future poet laureate, Alfred Austin, caught the mood of the hour in one couplet which became famous for the depth of bathos it plumbed. He wrote:

> Flash'd from his bed, the electric tidings came,
> He is not better; he is much the same.

A fellow guest, Lord Chesterfield, died, and Edward's condition became so grave and desperate that his doctors privately abandoned hope.

The approach of the tenth anniversary of his father's death on 14 December heightened the nation's sense of impending doom, and on 11 December the Queen was told Edward would not last the night.

In fact, the following morning saw an improvement, with the patient talking incessantly, and whistling and singing between bouts of laboured breathing.

On 14 December 'the crisis' or turning point of the disease occurred, and an exhausted prince slept like a baby.

Edward's battle with typhoid proved to be critical in more ways than one. With the Queen's persistent and unpopular withdrawal from public life following her husband's death, together with public disquiet at the profligate lifestyle led by Edward, Prince of Wales, there had been growing murmurings about republicanism. But the elemental upsurge of loyal emotions following the heir's brush with death—plus some astute politicking by William Gladstone, the Prime Minister—saw the nascent anti-monarchist ideas squashed.

Disease can sometimes have effects far beyond those observed in the individual.

Before we leave Sir James Clark we should mention a famous—and odd—case he attended 22 years before Prince Albert's demise. It concerned a member of the royal household and not—mercifully as we shall see—a royal personage.

At the beginning of 1839, when Clark had been Physician-in-Ordinary for only a couple of years, one of the Duchess of Kent's ladies-in-waiting, 32-year-old Lady Flora Hastings, was returning to London from a holiday in Scotland. A single, unchaperoned lady, she happened to be sharing the post-chaise with Sir John Conroy, Comptroller of the Duchess's household, a well-known lady's man. Lady Flora had been feeling ill over Christmas and was concerned about some bloating of the stomach.

Back in London she consulted Dr James Clark. Some compounds were prescribed, but later Clark indiscreetly commented they would be of little use as the lady may well be pregnant. On account of the long carriage trip with Conroy, this was also an ungracious suspicion entertained by the Duchess and the Prime Minister, Lord Melbourne. The court was full of gossip and there were dark hints about the somewhat scandalous travel arrangements. The Queen questioned Clark directly about the matter, and when he was hesitant in his answers, she confided to her diary that '. . . she is—to use plain language—*with child*!!' It was as though she had written an obscenity.

James Clark rightly but belatedly concluded the time had come for a fuller physical examination than had hitherto been performed. He resolved to investigate his 'patient's body with her stays removed', as he bluntly put it. Lady Flora cried 'infamy' and point-blank refused such an invasion of privacy. She did, however, relent some days later, doubtless after pressure from elsewhere.

One of the court's 'super specialists' was brought in: gynaecologist Sir Charles Clarke, who found the mortified lady to be *virgo intacta* and that there were no grounds for thinking a pregnancy could be implicated. The Queen was informed, was relieved and sent an apology, but rather uncharitably confided to her diary that she thought a virgin pregnancy may still be possible.

The still young and inexperienced James Clark hesitated about what to do next, a state of mind which may have been influenced by the fact that the relationship between Victoria and her mother the Duchess of Kent, never cordial, had taken a turn for the worse during the Flora Hastings scandal. The Duchess felt that Clark had cast an unjustified slur on the good lady—her hand-picked lady-in-waiting—and promptly dismissed the doctor from her service. But it was not her job to hire and fire royal doctors so Clark remained at court, doubtless trying to keep a low profile. Indeed, Lady Flora's family wrote a long letter of pained remonstration to the Queen, rightly naming Dr Clark as among those responsible for the public airing of the scandal.

The scandal, however, came to nothing, for as the weeks passed it became obvious that Lady Flora Hastings was dying. She lost weight, but retained her swollen abdomen which was now, with her skeletal appearance, more obvious than ever. She died on her 33rd birthday, 5 July 1839. A post-mortem showed her swelling was due to a 'cancerous tumour of the liver'. Primary cancer of the liver is in fact rare, so in hindsight it was more likely to have been a secondary tumour in the liver arising from a cancer elsewhere in the abdomen—perhaps the bowel or maybe ovary. We shall never know for certain, but even if it had been correctly diagnosed, a cure was beyond any of Lady Flora's medical advisers.

The ageing Sir James Clark retired as Physician-in-Ordinary to the royal household in 1862, not long after the death of the Prince Consort, and was succeeded by Sir William Jenner. Born in 1815 and a graduate of University College, London, Jenner's big claim to fame was that in 1851 he recognised the difference between two distinct but similarly named diseases: typhoid and typhus. Both are serious conditions, but caused by quite different bacteria. Typhoid is a water-borne disease, passed on via infected drinking water that has usually been contaminated by leaking sewage; typhus (or spotted fever) is a malady transmitted by lice, and common in, for instance, trench warfare, where lice are living on men who are in close proximity to one another.

Jenner had already been called in by Clark to help treat Prince Albert's typhoid. With Clark gone, and having met Jenner under harrowing circumstances, the Queen found Jenner's kindly, honest, good-humoured character and lack of pretence appealing and he got the top job. He lasted until succeeded by Sir James Reid in 1889.

Reid was interesting in that he left a diary and copious notes about his time in the royal household. Another Scotsman, he was born in 1849 in Aberdeenshire, north-east Scotland. His father was the local doctor in the town of Ellon. A bright boy at school, he progressed to Aberdeen Medical School at the age of nineteen, graduating top of the class in 1872. He then went to work in London as a general physician, and though offered a partnership in the practice he elected to take a post in Vienna. He did not know it at the time, but this would prove to be a highly fortuitous move that would change his life: while he was there he became fluent in German, a language that was still extensively used in the British royal court on account of both Victoria's and Albert's German relatives.

Reid left Vienna in 1877 with a glowing reference and returned to northeast Scotland to work in a country practice. He did his house calls to outlying farms and cottages on a Highland pony, and did so until April 1881, when out of the blue came the turning point of his life. Queen Victoria was looking for a successor to her retiring Resident Medical Attendant. She stipulated that he must be a Scotsman, preferably a native of her beloved Aberdeenshire, well-qualified medically—and, crucially, conversant in German. Reid had many relatives and friends in Aberdeenshire, so his name was soon put forward. The Queen interviewed him and recorded in her journal that Dr Reid came with the very highest testimonials, and that he appealed because of his shrewdness, tact, honesty and good humour.

So on 8 July 1881, at the age of only 31, James Reid started as the Queen's Resident Medical Attendant. In 1889, he became a Physician-Extraordinary whereupon the old Queen wrote, '. . . there is no more physician in whom I had more confidence than Doctor Reid'. He remained in his post until Victoria died in 1901; he then became Physician-in-Ordinary to King Edward VII. On Edward's death in 1911 he was appointed Physician-in-Ordinary to the new King, George V. Sir James Reid died in 1923.

But let us go back a few years. Sir James Reid's habit of keeping a diary has been mentioned, and he is now perhaps best remembered for the detail he left, firstly, of Queen Victoria's illnesses, and more especially her death, and secondly, the secret mission he had been commanded to carry out on Queen Victoria's death. (Extracts of his diary have been published by his granddaughter-in-law, Michaela Reid, in her fascinating book *Ask Sir James*.)

As we have said, Victoria could be a difficult patient. A great believer in fresh air, she ordered that all the palace windows be left open in all weathers. She forbade open fires, and in winter rooms were often filled with a swirling icy mist. The Queen's main complaints were chronic indigestion—brought on, Reid commented, by large helpings of suet pudding of which she was very fond—and rheumatism, producing pains in her legs and back, which towards the end of her life forced her into a wheelchair; opaque cataracts and a chronic anxiety state rounded off her medical history. After the death of 'Dear Albert' in 1861, she became a recluse and experienced long periods of teary depression and unresolved anxiety, in the end becoming a demanding, manipulative and creative invalid.

As the new Resident Medical Attendant, Reid had to help stave off Her Majesty's descent into day-long anxiety. He saw her three or four times a day, every day, and whenever summoned, day or night, to hear her recount her fears and ruminate on her sins. Remarkably, despite his medical attentiveness, Sir James never physically examined the regal personage. (Nowadays this would be regarded as criminal negligence, but in the exaggerated modesty characteristic of the Victorian era, it was the accepted practice.) So, in his twenty years of service, he never saw Victoria in her bed, as she always sat in a chair fully dressed, even during the night. The first time he actually viewed her lying down beneath the sheets was on 16 January 1901, six days before she died of a cerebral haemorrhage.

A few years earlier, in February 1898, the Queen had spoken to Reid about what she wished to be done on her death, and handed to him two memoranda. These had been written years before in 1875. One had become redundant because it stated she wished her 'devoted personal attendant and true friend John Brown' be near at hand on her death, but he had died in 1883, so this was now not possible. The second note gave rambling instructions on what the family and her attending physician were required to do on Victoria's death. It was incumbent on Sir James Reid to carry out this latter instruction.

When the old Queen died she was undressed, and for the first time ever her personal doctor observed her naked. To his great surprise he saw that she had a ventral hernia and prolapse. The ventral hernia was a great bulge in the abdominal wall due to weakness of the abdominal muscles, probably a result of multiple pregnancies, given that she had been delivered of nine children. The prolapse was a falling of the uterus or womb down the vagina. There are several grades of this disability, from a minor descent, to one progressing through the vagina, to complete externalisation of the organ. (Nowadays it is eminently treatable by surgery and is certainly not common, but at that time curative surgery with crude anaesthesia was regarded too great a hazard.) In his diaries Reid did not comment on the magnitude of the prolapse, but Her Majesty's troublesome displacement—which she found far too embarrassing to mention even to her medical adviser—must have been rather severe to have been on view for him to see it.

While it was still in her bedchamber, Victoria's body was washed, then dressed in a white satin dressing-gown. Over the gown was placed the brilliant-blue ribbon of the Order of the Garter, and the star of the Order was attached to the gown. She was then laid into the coffin. Numerous other memorabilia were put in the casket, such as photographs, the Prince Consort's dressing-gown, children's embroidery and some flowers. The care of the Queen's person was Reid's responsibility until the coffin was sealed, and as the maids fussed about putting in the various bric-a-brac, he quietly approached the body from the left side, intent on fulfilling the secret charge laid out by his employer three years before.

He quietly moved aside the flowers nestling in Victoria's left hand, which had been sent by the new queen, Alexandra. In her left hand he placed a photograph of John Brown and a lock of his hair, which Reid himself had wrapped in tissue paper. (The Queen had stipulated the left hand, possibly as it was nearer the heart.) He also put a second wedding ring on one of her fingers. The first was her original ring given by Prince Albert on their marriage; the second had been given to her years before by John Brown, and had belonged to his mother.

It is not known whether the Queen and John Brown had a sexual relationship. There is no doubt they were close and that he spoke very directly to her—occasionally in a gruff, almost denigrating and rude, manner that no-one else at Court would dare to use. More than that is pure speculation; nonetheless that ring provides intriguing circumstantial evidence.

Having completed his charge, the doctor rearranged the sheaf of blooms and casually moved away, his act of homage unobserved by others in the room.

The royal family then came to view the body. None knew of the deposition placed in the obscured left hand by the faithful and discreet doctor, and Queen Victoria carried her secret to the grave.

7

Hitler's doctor

Dr Theodor Gilbert Morell became Adolf Hitler's personal physician at the end of 1936, a position he retained until the end of World War II. He spent the dying days of the Third Reich in the Berlin bunker, and left at Hitler's request just before his Führer suicided on 30 April 1945. He made his way to the airport to catch one of the last planes out of the beleaguered city, leaving behind a quantity of pre-prepared medicines which were subsequently administered by Hitler's valet, presumably in the vain hope the Führer would somehow escape.

When he left the bunker, Morell prudently made for the Allied lines, where he was picked up by the Americans to become Prisoner 21672. He was interned at the American civilian internment camp, which had previously been the infamous Dachau concentration camp. Though questioned, Morell was never charged with war crimes; he was later released and passed into history. A grossly obese man who suffered from a speech impediment that may have been due to a previous cerebrovascular accident, he died in the German lakeside resort of Tegernsee in May 1948, aged 61.

But let us go back a few years to the doctor's halcyon days. Morell was born in 1886 in a small village in Upper Hesse, the son of a schoolmaster. He read medicine at Heidelberg and later studied at Grenoble, Paris and Munich, where he obtained a PhD, his thesis being on treating the transverse lie of the foetus during pregnancy. His medical degree and licence to practise was issued by the Bavarian State in 1913, and after graduation he did a few trips as a ship's medical officer and later served as an army medical officer on the Western Front during World War I.

In 1920 he married Hannelore Moller, a wealthy actress, and became a general practitioner in Berlin, where he was regarded as an unconventional physician for his use of holistic and alternative therapies. This seemed to attract high-society patients, and his practice was mainly drawn from the world of theatre and film. These trendy contacts led to offers of posts as private physician from the Shah of Persia and the King of Romania, among other luminaries.

Being of a somewhat Jewish appearance, in 1933 he thought it prudent to join the Nazi party and moved to a more prestigious area of the German capital, where he called himself a venereologist. It was as a practitioner in this specialty that in 1936 he treated professional photographer Heinrich Hoffmann for gonorrhoea. Although he did not know it at the time, the meeting was to change his life.

Hoffmann's assistant was Eva Braun, then aged 26 and, since 1932, Adolf Hitler's mistress. She took a shine to Morell and, with Hoffman in tow, Braun introduced Morell to Hitler—though not, as far as we know, because the leader was suffering from a venereal disease, which his addled mind associated only with the Jewish race. Eva Braun instead thought the doctor could cure her lover's recurrent and socially embarrassing chronic intestinal gas problems with his alternative medicines. Morell said he could cure the Chancellor within a year, and on the strength of that promise was appointed Hitler's personal physician. Morell's wife, however, was not happy with his new post.

Since the early 1930s Hitler had experienced cramping pains in his right upper abdomen. They occurred shortly after meals, and he commonly had to leave the table so as not to embarrass his guests with his symptoms. The pains waxed and waned and were located in the region of the gall bladder. Later in 1941 the pain became quite severe and was accompanied by vomiting. In September 1944, he had a bout of jaundice. In between times he suffered from abdominal distension and was not above passing intestinal gas from both ends of the alimentary tract at socially inappropriate moments. After one of their meetings, Mussolini is reported to have had all the windows thrown open to dispel the fetid smell.

The story sounds very like gall bladder disease, with stones causing intermittent obstruction of the bile flow, leading to jaundice. Regrettably, no report on the status of the gall bladder has come down to us from the Russian pathologist who did a post-mortem on the Führer after the end of the war.

For the symptoms Morell prescribed a battery of preparations, including Dr Koster's anti-gas pills, which contained strychnine, belladonna and gentian; pills of ox bile, papaverine (an alkaloid derived from opium which relaxes muscles of the gut) and, paradoxically in the circumstances, capsules containing yeast, and Mutaflor, a capsule of living *E. coli* bacteria. Oddly enough, improvement was noticed.

Flushed with success, the Morells became a part of Hitler's inner social circle. The doctor added more therapies; most, such as extract of the seminal vesicles and prostate of an ox, were of little therapeutic value, though on account of their male hormonal content Eva Braun may have thought otherwise. Conversely, in 1937 Hitler was also given Progynon B, an oral preparation of oestradiol and hydroxyprogesterone, female sex hormones.

As Hitler's physician, Morell was recommended to other high-fliers in the Nazi party, but most dismissed him as a quack, or at least an opportunist. Herman Goering called Morell 'The Reich Injection Master or Impresario'. Another called him 'The Master of the Imperial Needle'. All nicknames imply the overuse of drug injections. Eventually he even fell out of favour with Eva Braun.

Other medications Morell used were distinctly dangerous. These included cocaine eye drops that contained enough drugs to cause psychotic behaviour, and Dr Morell's special chocolate-coated, gold-wrapped 'Vitamultin' tablets, a concoction of caffeine and methyl amphetamine given routinely as a morning stimulant. Morell never told anyone (including the Führer) what he was administering, except to say they were vitamins or naturally occurring ingredients.

What Morell was never able to treat were the outrageous outbursts of temper and feelings of paranoia from which his boss suffered. Never an even-tempered man, Hitler's seriously psychotic outbursts became even more ferocious after 1942 when the Russian campaign was beginning to falter.

After an unsuccessful attempt on his life on 20 July 1944, Hitler merely suffered bruising of the elbow and knee after being thrown against a door frame. He also ruptured both eardrums. They were healed by September. For his superficial wounds, Morell treated him with penicillin ointment. This had only very recently been released to the US Army for testing, so where he acquired it is a mystery. When interrogated after the war he claimed ignorance of the fact.

I wonder how much of Adolf Hitler's bizarre paranoia and grotesque mindset was as much due to these treatments as his psychotic personality?

8

Stalin's doctors

Josef Vissarionovich Djugashvili was born in Georgia, Russia, in 1879. Had he retained that name he may well have lived and died a peasant. But he didn't, for in 1912 he changed it to the Russian for 'man of steel'—Josef Stalin. It suited him well.

Stalin was born into abject poverty, the son of a drunken, abusive shoemaker. He was educated at a local theological seminary, from which he was expelled for 'propagating Marxism'. As a child he endured a severe attack of smallpox which left his face permanently scarred. He was so disfigured that when he came to power, thousands of photographs had to be doctored to disguise the unsightly lesions.

At the age of ten his left arm was injured, possibly as a result of being thrashed by his father. The bone became infected, causing osteomyelitis. Poor treatment by an unknown doctor led to a 'Volkmann's contracture', where the arm muscles are permanently contracted, the hand will not open fully and muscle control is lost. There was also a permanent shortening of the arm of about 7.5 centimetres. He often wore a glove, allegedly for rheumatism, but probably to conceal the disability. At times he also wore a brace on the arm, as can be seen in some unguarded photographed moments.

Despite these defects, Stalin was physically very strong, as illustrated by the story that late in life he swung the beefy Marshal Tito off his feet in a bear hug.

But his upbringing had its effect, for as the years rolled by Stalin grew more and more paranoid, suspicious of even those close to him. In fits of this mental disturbance he had thousands shot on the suspicion of plotting against him; his motorcade comprised five identical cars which changed position continually to confuse would-be assassins. In his apartment there were four rooms fitted out as bedrooms, and not before retiring did he choose the one in which to sleep. This man was obviously seriously affected by his mental illness—bad enough in an ordinary citizen, but catastrophic for someone in absolute power and whose temper was feared by those about him. Stalin was in charge with an iron grip, and with his security guards and his well-planned lifestyle, there was little chance of getting away with a coup to unseat him as Secretary General of the Communist Party.

After World War II, however, Stalin was forced into partial retirement due to high blood pressure, whereupon he became even more suspicious, calculating and irritable. Locks and bolts increased in number around his house, and he had members of the Politburo eat with him every night so he knew where they were. All his food had to be tasted, and often had to be doubly tested by his cronies.

By 1952 he was dosing himself with a variety of pills and iodine drops for unspecified symptoms. Though he had a physician—several in fact—Stalin had become so paranoid that he considered it far too dangerous to let them near enough to properly examine him. The doctors knew what was the best course for them to follow if they wanted to keep not only their job, but possibly their lives as well.

Then, for reasons unknown, Stalin's dark thoughts about his doctors escalated and he was able to give vent to his worst suspicions when, out of the blue on 13 January 1953, the official newspaper *Pravda* proclaimed the leader had uncovered a sinister medical conspiracy.

It seems the dictator had received a letter from a Dr Lydia Timashuk, who was not one of his inner medical entourage and from all accounts was a medical nonentity. In it she claimed Comrade Andrei Zhdanov and other Soviet luminaries had been poisoned by Stalin's doctors some years before.

An able man, Zhdanov had been the party chief in Leningrad and freely canvassed as Stalin's successor. It seems Georgy Malenkov, the deputy prime minister stationed in Moscow, coveted this top post, and Zhdanov's death in 1948 was suspiciously providential as far as Malenkov's aspirations were concerned. (Indeed, in the end, on Stalin's death, Malenkov did get the job as de facto party leader, until forced to resign in February 1955 when Nikita Khrushchev secured the permanent position.)

Following his old philosophy that 'if a report is 10 per cent true we should regard the entire report as fact', Stalin believed the letter: after all, he was in the right frame of mind to believe tell of any medical plot. The Leningrad

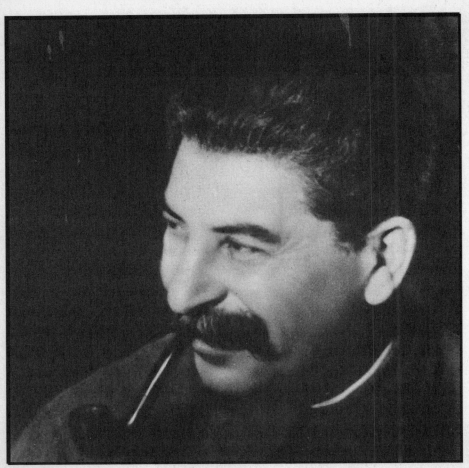

Josef Stalin

Communist Party mastermind had, of course, been treated by allegedly trusted Kremlin doctors who were well known and respected in the medical world, though perhaps to a lesser extent in the political world.

Anyway, the hint was enough. Nine of Stalin's doctors were arrested and jailed for what came to be known as the 'Doctors' Plot'. Among those who got the dread knock on the door was Stalin's personal physician of twenty years, the thoroughly trustworthy Dr V.N. Vinogradov. He was arrested, beaten, manacled and committed to a dungeon on the suspicion of being a British spy.

Significantly, six of the doctors arrested had Jewish surnames. It was said in the charges that five had worked for American intelligence through a Jewish organisation, and three were British agents. All were distinguished in the medical field, but anti-Semitism was in the air.

More letters poured in purporting medical involvement in a dastardly intrigue and Stalin allowed the press campaign to gain momentum. Members of the Presidium—a permanent committee that acts when the legislature is in recess—felt there was a lack of substance in the accusations, but never discussed their doubts openly, because, as Khrushchev was to write later, 'once Stalin had made up his mind and started to deal with a problem, there wasn't anything to do'.

The interrogations began. Stalin was in a rage and Khrushchev reports that the Soviet leader berated the Minister of State Security to 'throw the doctors in chains, beat them to a pulp and grind them into powder'.

All the doctors confessed. Who wouldn't?

On 20 January 1953 Dr Timashuk was awarded the Order of Lenin for her denunciations, which were regarded as a significant act of public service.

On 4 April, a month after Stalin's death, the honour was revoked by his slightly more conciliatory successor, and that same day the seven remaining living doctors were released. Two had been tortured to death.

Turning now to the leader's death. On 1 March 1953, Stalin had a stroke. At first his fearful servants were loath to disturb their apparently sleeping chief, but when they realised what had happened, all hell broke loose and his room was suddenly packed with a host of doctors, politicians and security men.

There was no public announcement of any illness until three days later, 4 March. Then Radio Moscow gave the news that Comrade Stalin had lost consciousness, was unable to speak, and his right leg and arm were paralysed. Nine doctors were in attendance—a group of men who, I am sure, harboured very mixed feelings about their futures, especially as they saw the parlous medical state to which their chief had descended.

The communiqué added that the Secretary General's treatment was under the constant surveillance of the Central Committee of the Communist Party and the Soviet Government. In reality Stalin's chances of recovery were slim, but such guidance by a committee of men with axes to grind would have snuffed out any hope.

Over the next few hours a wealth of medical detail was given to show that everything possible was being done. Thus oxygen was given for the irregular and gasping Cheyne–Stokes respiration, with camphor, caffeine, strophanthin and penicillin being administered, and leeches being applied to the head. An artificial respirator was trundled in, but, as nobody could work it, the machine lay idle in the corner as the patient slowly choked to death.

He died on 5 March 1953, aged 73.

A fully reported post-mortem absolved the attendant medical men from blame. Nevertheless, of the nine doctors who signed the report, one died suddenly six weeks later, and two others were removed from their posts and disappeared forever shortly afterwards.

The Doctors' Plot was Stalin's last purge. As it stopped suddenly on 24 February, it has been postulated that from that date Stalin was too ill to carry on directing affairs. It has been claimed the stroke actually occurred on that day and that there was a power vacuum until his reported death on 5 March.

It has also been mooted that Stalin was murdered by poison given by a person or persons unknown, and that the battery of terrorised doctors went along with the lie. To support the suggestion that there was also outside non-medical interference, it has been pointed out that after the first bulletin, the subsequent communiqués became more woolly and less medically correct—for instance, the albumen and red cell ratio in the urine was said to be normal. It is a redundant statement as in the normal course of events they are never present.

We shall never know.

Stalin had shown mental instability for years, and in his time ordered purges during which thousands died. He finally turned on the doctors—but if the dictator had died three months earlier they would have been spared and this tale never told.

PART II

Doctors in the Arts

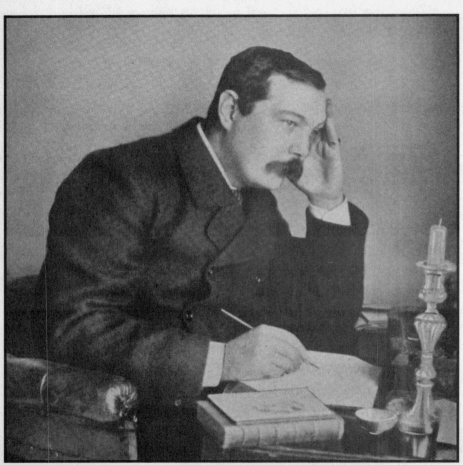

Arthur Conan Doyle

9

Two early rabble-rousers: François Rabelais and Girolamo Fracastoro

These two rather rumbustious and graceless—though articulate—fifteenth-century physicians-cum-authors were almost exact contemporaries. The more famous, François Rabelais, was born in a farmhouse in Chinon, France, around 1494, and Girolamo Fracastoro in Verona, Italy, a little earlier, around 1483. It is thought they both died in the same year, 1553. Each made their mark on literature more than medicine, and each was famous in their own lifetime, albeit for different reasons.

François Rabelais (c. 1494–1553)

Rabelais was by profession a physician, but by conviction a writer, and it is as such he is remembered today, perhaps because he has become such a byword as a purveyor of coarse, boisterous humour and satire. So much so, in fact, that the description of such offerings have passed into the language as being Rabelaisian.

Confusion surrounds his birth date, but consensus among the literati is that it was either in 1493 or 1494. His father was both a lawyer and apothecary, and at the age of nine young François was sent to the Benedictine abbey of Seuilly, and from there he was transferred to a Franciscan monastery near Angers in western France on the River Maine. He became a novice in the Franciscan order and entered the monastery of Fontenay-le-Comte, where he had access to a great library. It was here he learned Greek, Hebrew and Arabic, as well as, of course, Latin and French. Added to this academic load, he learned about botany, astronomy and lastly medicine.

While in Orders in the early days of the Renaissance he attained a reputation as a talker and thinker, and was able to disseminate some of his views—at least to those who could read, mainly clerics—via the new-fangled invention of printing. But his readily expressed and forceful views were not welcome among the monastery hierarchy and he left under a cloud, to finish his studies in a Benedictine house near Orléans on the River Loire in central France.

As a mature-aged student, in 1530 Rabelais enrolled in the great and ancient medical school at Montpellier: the university in southern France that was founded in 1289. He must have had friends in high places, for instead of the usual two years, it took him just six weeks to receive his bachelor degree in medicine. He went on to work in a hospital in Lyon, and seven years later obtained his full doctorate, or MD.

Rabelais was inhibited in his work as a surgeon as his ordination precluded him from using the scalpel or practising for gain. But what he could and did do was write, using his literary skill as a therapeutic tool by creating laughter—the best medicine. Though we may consider his offerings uncouth, they were in fact couched in the everyday language of his time.

In 1532, while working in the hospital in Lyon, there appeared at a local fair a book, *The Great and Inestimable Chronicles of the Grand and Enormous Giant Gargantua*. Though commonly ascribed to Rabelais, the pundits think he almost certainly did not write it—but he did write and publish in the same year a sequel which is now regarded his first masterpiece, *Pantagruel*, 'king of the thirsty ones' or Dipsodes. Part serious, part nonsense, it depicts the birth, education and exploits of the giant Pantagruel, and was assured success by being suppressed as obscene by the Sorbonne University in Paris. As an example of its alleged 'obscenity', Pantagruel regarded the codpiece as the principal piece of military equipment, for 'when a man loses his head only the individual perishes; but if the balls were lost, the whole human race would die out'. Perhaps mild by our standards, but sacrilegious then.

Spurred on by ridicule, in 1534 Rabelais brought out his second and more famous ribald satire, a new *Gargantua*, father of Pantagruel, who was another giant and more full of both sense and wisdom than Pantagruel. The word has passed into the language, gargantuan meaning enormous, and usually applied to appetite. Both books were published under the pseudonym Alcofri bas Nasier—which is a very contrived anagram of François Rabelais—and both books enjoyed great success.

In his book *Gargantua* he satirises the medical profession, having the giant born by entering a hollow vein and climbing through the diaphragm to a point above the shoulders where the vein divides in two. He takes the left fork coming out of the left ear and immediately cries, 'Give me a drink! Drink! Drink!' Later, when sent to Paris, he picked up the bells of Notre Dame to hang round a horse's neck.

When his son Pantagruel is about to be born, there first came down the birth canal 68 mule drivers, with each mule loaded with salt; nine dromedaries loaded with hams; seven camels loaded with eels; and finally 24 cartloads of leeks, garlic, onions and shallots. Rather superfluously the writer added that all this frightened the midwives. Later Pantagruel thought of becoming a doctor, but decided against it because physicians smelt of suppositories, 'like old devils'.

They don't write books like that nowadays: authors lack such fertile imaginations.

While in Lyon Rabelais not only wrote these classics but also found time to edit several medical textbooks which were of a somewhat more serious nature.

After he gained his full doctorate of medicine in 1537, Rabelais taught at Montpellier Medical School, which along with the schools in Paris, and in Padua and Bologna in Italy, was one of the supreme European centres of medical learning during the Middle Ages. He only stayed for about a year, then re-entered the Church to become personal physician/priest to the French ambassador to the Vatican, and also to several cardinals.

In 1546 he published his third book, this time under his own name. Again the Sorbonne condemned it (surely that alone would have ensured more heavy sales), so he fled to the town of Metz in the Lorraine region of France, where he worked as a general physician.

He left to become a demonstrator in anatomy at Lyons, where his remarkable scholarship—especially in botany, pharmacy (rabelaisin is a glycoside that he discovered in the plant *Lophopetalum toxicum*) and his grasp of anatomy—was marvelled over. He continued to publish, and even anticipated the microscope by 100 years when he described sperm as being 'like a hundred carpenters' nails'.

He only practised medicine for nine years, but was said in that time to have described treating fractures of the thigh by continuous extension, and strangulated hernias by incising them using a syringe with a concealed blade.

In 1547 he was summoned to Rome to act as physician to a newly appointed cardinal from France, whom he had treated in the past. He worked in this rather plum job for two years, during which he had time to bring out another book. It was the third book in the Gargantua–Pantagruel series, called simply *Le Tiers Livre*. This one was banned by the theologians.

The uninhibited riotous mirth and licence with which Rabelais wrote made him many enemies in high places, but to us 500 years on they are a treasury of wit, wisdom and above all satire. He was one of the greatest and certainly funniest French writers of the sixteenth century. From the high-level medical posts he filled, especially in the Church, he must have been no mean doctor either.

He died in 1553. His unauthenticated but pertinent last words are said to have been, 'Draw the curtain, the farce is over.'

Girolamo Fracastoro (c. 1483–1553)

Our next subject is better known as Hieronymus Fracastorius, but is less well known outside the medical profession than François Rabelais. He was born in Verona, Italy, in either 1478 or 1483, into the family of a nobleman. Two circumstances of his infancy are remarkable. First it is said that when born his mouth was so small that it was necessary to enlarge it with a surgical instrument so he could suckle. Second, while in the arms of his mother, she was struck by a bolt of lightning which killed her, while the infant was unharmed. Both events are so remarkable as to be exceedingly unlikely to have happened. I am sure the fable has been passed down the years like a Chinese whisper in that the details have grown out of all proportion to the truth.

A bright child, Fracastorius went to the greatest medical school of the era at Padua, near Venice, where he studied not just medicine but philosophy, mathematics and *belles lettres*. After graduation he went into private practice as a physician and had a special interest in epidemic diseases. He fairly quickly gained a reputation as a diagnostician, and his renown spread throughout Italy and into Europe. Despite being a busy practitioner, he found time to study music, geography, botany and especially poetry, the publication of which led to his general fame.

In 1546 he wrote *On the Contagion and Contagious Diseases (De Contagione)*, which had a modern ring about it because it expressed the concept of bacterial infections, then quite unknown. He also concluded that infection was caused by imperceptibly small particles, or 'seeds' as he called them, not perceived by our senses and passed on by contact both through a human intermediary or by means of fomites such as lice. He also gave the first clear account of typhus.

He showed considerable clinical nous, but his work was largely ignored until Louis Pasteur came along with his 'germ theory' towards the end of the nineteenth century, some 350 years later. By right Fracastorius should be regarded as the founder of modern epidemiology, but he gained considerably more fame as a writer, especially after his long Virgilian masterpiece *Syphilis Sive Morbus Gallicus*. For it was he who gave the great and rapidly spreading scourge 'syphilis' its name, though he himself called it the French disease. Six years after his death in 1553, a statue was erected in Verona, embellished with a chiselled eulogy to the author of 'that divine poem, *Syphilis*'.

Not known in ancient Egypt or in Biblical times, the first real evidence of the malady was discovered in the twentieth century in skeletons from the mid-fourteenth century uncovered in the ruins of a monastery in Hull, Eastern England. However, it is generally accepted that syphilis was first recorded in 1493.

It first manifest itself in any large number among French and Neapolitan soldiers and their mercenaries during the siege of Naples by the French in 1495. As the military made its way home, it quickly spread through Europe, and each country blamed another for its origin: the French called it the Italian disease, the English the French pox, the Germans blamed the French (*malade Frankzos*), and Spain and Poland also received dishonourable mention.

But what was Fracastorius' poetic masterpiece about?

Fracastorius himself claims it was written in one of his lighter moments, and implies the disease originated from the exploratory voyages of Columbus to Central America. *Syphilis Sive Morbus Gallicus* first appeared in 1530, 35 or so years after that event, and he dedicated it to his old friend and classmate from Padua days, Cardinal Bembo.

The epic poem relates to a legend of the shepherd Syphilis, who lived on one of the isles in the West Indies (the Spanish Main) and whose job it was to look after the animal stock of the local ruler, King Alcithous. In an act of impiety the youth was struck by the French disease. It is a very long piece, but here are some of the relevant extracts. It starts:

> A shepherd once (distrust not ancient fame),
> Possest these downs and Syphilis was his name,
> A Thousand heifers in these vales he fed,
> A thousand ewes to those fair rivers led.

It goes on that the youth broke the rules and erected an altar to his monarch rather than to the sun god, Apollo. The god was understandably displeased and the poem menacingly records, 'all seeing sun no longer could sustain these practices, but with enrag'd Disdain Darts forth such pestilent malignant Beams' and 'shed infection on Air, Earth and Streams'.

The hapless shepherd boy was the first to suffer from the divine wrath, and the event is beautifully described (buboes are enlarged and infected lymph glands):

> He first wore buboes dreadful to the sight,
> Felt strange pains and sleepless past the night:
> From him the malady received its name,
> The neighbouring shepherds catcht the spreading flame;
> At last in city and court was known,
> And seized ambitious on his throne.

Treatment by mercury and guaiacum or Holy Wood, a remedy of West Indian origin, also gets a mention. Mercury became the standard treatment in Europe from the early sixteenth century until the early twentieth century.

Fracastorius' epic was contemporaneously regarded as a masterpiece, and syphilis soon became the universal term for the disease. The poem was translated into English about 100 years later by Irishman Nahum Tate, who became poet laureate in 1692, but whose real and only claim to fame was that he wrote the Christmas carol 'While Shepherds Watch Their Flocks by Night'. I wonder if he gained inspiration from Fracastorius and his pox-ridden shepherd boy, Syphilis?

10

Sometime doctor and Irish genius: Oliver Goldsmith

On 21 August 1766, Sir Joshua Reynolds completed a portrait of a London doctor. It showed a man with a prominent nose, hooded eyes and a forehead creased with worry, maybe wonder, maybe surprise that he had come so far up the social ladder. It hangs now in Woburn Abbey in Bedfordshire, England. Few of its present-day admirers connect the sitter with being the failed medical practitioner or the high-stake gambler that he was; they only know him to be the Irish genius Oliver Goldsmith (1728–1774), one of the literary giants of the eighteenth century.

Son of the curate in the parish of Kilkenny West, Goldsmith was born on 10 November 1728 in Passamore, County Longford, at his grandmother's substantial, but unpretentious, farmhouse, Smith Hill. He was the youngest of four children in a household where the total income was £40 a year, a sum which left precious little room for the frivolities of life. There would have been five children, but the eldest, Margery, died.

When Oliver was two, the parish parson died and his father, Charles Goldsmith, moved up the pecking order from curate to incumbent of the living. The family moved to the village of Lissoy and into a commodious residence boasting two storeys and five bay windows. Such windows were an indication that the occupant was a person of substance. (Some of the atmosphere of the village can be felt in Goldsmith's later masterpiece, *The Vicar of Wakefield*; the opening line of his consummate poem 'The Deserted Village'—'Sweet Auburn! Loveliest village of the plain'—is regarded as a highly idealised portrait of Lissoy.)

As a youth Oliver Goldsmith was a rabble-rouser and gambler who retained a fragile relationship with sobriety. Nonetheless, he was bright enough to gain admission to Trinity College, Dublin, with a view to following his father into the Church, but the idea had scant appeal to him. He decided to try his luck in America, but got no further than the departure port of Cork.

His father then set him up with £50 to study law in London. This time he got as far as Dublin, where he promptly gambled away his allowance. Studying medicine was thought to be the answer of last resort by an exasperated Rev. Goldsmith, so Oliver was packed off to Edinburgh, arriving at the famed medical school in 1752. There he was more noted for his social gifts and drinking prowess than any academic application, although he was alleged to have drawn some inspiration from his highly regarded anatomy professor, Alexander Monro.

(In passing, a century or so later this mentor became known as Alexander Monro 'Primus' to distinguish him from his son and grandson, three men who succeeded each other to the Chair of Anatomy. As these latter two were also both called Alexander, down the track they became known as Alexander Monro 'Secundus' and Alexander Monro 'Tertius'. Between them the dynasty occupied the Chair of Anatomy for 126 years from 1720 to 1846.)

After two years at Edinburgh, Goldsmith became restless and decided to finish his medical studies in Paris or Leiden, presumably to be nearer to where his kind of boisterous action was at.

Neither university suited his free spirit and he wandered Europe, mainly on foot, living on his wits and earning an occasional night's board and lodging as a flute-playing busker. He eventually fetched up in Padua, Italy. Although there is no doubt that he did attend this world-famous and ancient medical school situated about 50 kilometres from Venice, no record of his graduation exists. If he ever did get a medical degree, it must have been here, for he attended no more seats of learning after returning to London in 1756.

Back in England's capital penniless, Goldsmith set himself up as what he called 'a physician', and we would regard as a general practitioner. That was in Bankside, an unfashionable area in Southwark at the southern end of London Bridge, and—appropriately for a dubiously qualified practitioner—near to the Clink gaol.

The lack of a certificate was no impediment to such clinical aspirations in the 1700s. The services of Members of the College of Physicians were very expensive, and apothecaries were regarded as a cross between a pharmacist and a district nurse. Our hero fell between these two extremes and managed to write such bizarre prescriptions that, as the renowned painter Joshua Reynolds was later to record, apothecaries refused to make them up.

Business was slow and mainly comprised unreliable payers, such as local prostitutes and passing sailors, so Goldsmith had enough spare time to moonlight as a proofreader for Samuel Richardson, one of the founders of the modern English novel, whose well-known early works include such classics as *Pamela* and *Clarissa, or, The History of a Young Lady*.

The move was pivotal to his future aspirations, for by now Goldsmith himself was doing some writing, which the great Richardson favourably reviewed.

Despite this, the doctor-cum-author seemed doomed to be an impoverished failure. Then he met the publisher of the *Monthly Review*, who was taken by the doctor's Irish wit and style and invited him to contribute to the magazine. In 1758 there appeared his first definitive work, a translation of the *Memoirs of Jean Marteilhe*, a persecuted French Protestant: he was on his way. His heart had never been in medical practice and, as he paid them scant attention, what clientele he had just withered away—and good riddance.

So within a year of arriving in London, Goldsmith had found his metier. In 1759 he started and edited a weekly publication, *The Bee*, and contributed to *The Busy Body* and *The Lady's Magazine*. At least he was making a bit of a name for himself as a writer as well as earning some money.

In May 1761 he met Dr Samuel Johnson. In 1764 Goldsmith was awarded the singular accolade of being invited to join as one of the nine original members of the celebrated literary gathering simply known as the Literary Club, of which Johnson was the presiding genius. It met at the Turk's Head Tavern, Gerrard Street. The meeting room is still there and is now a Chinese book shop.

In 1766 Goldsmith published his novel *The Vicar of Wakefield*, and his reputation as an author of some standing was secured. His medical background, however, was still held in some regard for, to his mortification, on one occasion his qualification came under critical scrutiny.

The story goes that in 1769, the Literary Club members were invited to Oxford. Here there was a courtesy in place whereby it was possible to convert a degree obtained elsewhere into an Oxford equivalent (*ad eundem gradum*). Goldsmith could not provide the necessary documentation, whereupon the club's alumni felt his claim to having a bachelor degree in Medicine was bogus—as indeed it may well have been. Still, that was no impediment to composing his poem 'The Deserted Village' in 1770, which I myself learned at school 170 years later, and parts of which I can still recite. In 1780, Goldsmith attained high dramatic honours with his play, *She Stoops to Conquer*.

Between 1772 and 1774 he suffered from dysuria (painful urination) and intermittent fever, probably due to bladder stones leading to severe infection of the kidneys. 'Dr' Goldsmith rejected the advice of several proper doctors, dosing himself with Dr James's Fever Powder, which was very popular at the time. Unfortunately the medication's main constituent was antimony, a highly toxic substance. As a result of imbibing it he went inexorably downhill, and finally died in April 1774.

Goldsmith was buried in the Temple Churchyard and the club erected a monument to him in Westminster Abbey. It is still there.

Whatever his other qualities, Goldsmith was a lousy doctor. He did, however, leave us a number of enduring literary riches, both poetry and prose, which are as highly regarded today as they were 250 years ago.

Though he never returned to Ireland, Goldsmith never forgot his roots, for he rightly knew that his early schooling there, coupled with the influence his countrymen had on his fertile imagination, had contributed substantially to his genius.

All his faults are such that one loves him still the better for them.
Oliver Goldsmith, *The Good-Natured Man*, 1768

11

Words most sublime: John Keats and Somerset Maugham

John Keats (1795–1821)

After having passed the examination of the Worshipful Society of Apothecaries of London on 25 July 1816 to become possibly its most famous licentiate ever, John Keats turned to poetry as his life's work. Tragically his life was to be short, but long enough for him to emerge as one of the greatest poets in the English language.

Keats was born in 1795, the eldest son of a livery stable-keeper, or ostler, in Enfield, north London. His father died in a riding accident in 1804, and his mother of tuberculosis four years later.

After his mother's death, Keats left school and became apprenticed to Thomas Hammond, a surgeon in Edmonton, Middlesex. He knew this post was to be followed by walking the wards at one or other of the country's teaching hospitals, most of which were situated in London. That was the method of entry into the profession up to about 1815, when a new Medical Act was promulgated and medical schools became the main teaching centres from the start of the course, while apprenticeships were phased out.

Initially he enjoyed the life in Edmonton and planned on becoming an

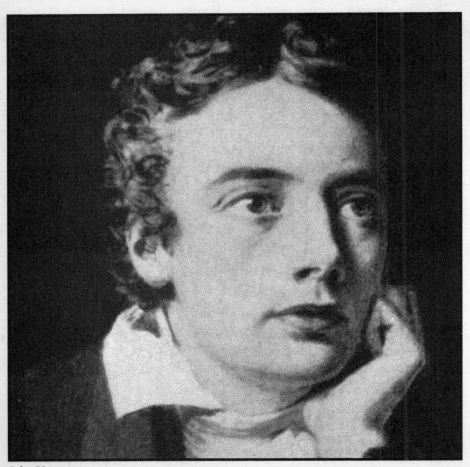

John Keats

apothecary or general practitioner, as the job was coming to be known. He lived above the surgeon's shop, spending his days grooming the horses, sweeping out the surgery, cleaning the medicine bottles and picking up medical tips on the way. But he left enough time to compose his first poem, 'Imitation of Spencer'.

In late 1814 Keats and Hammond quarrelled. Their relationship remained strained thereafter until 1 October 1815, when the youth registered as a student at Guy's Hospital, Southwark, on the south side of the Thames over London Bridge. It cost him 22 shillings to enrol and a further £25 to register as a surgical pupil for twelve months. At that time Guy's and St Thomas's Hospitals were joined and operated as one. They split in the mid-nineteenth century when construction of the new underground railway and London Bridge station managed to cut the two institutions in two. St Thomas's moved to Lambeth, where author Somerset Maugham was to study about 80 years later.

John Keats attended lectures given by, among others, Henry Cline, the pathologist/surgeon who famously described and treated the massive hydrocele of historian Edward Gibbon in the 1790s, and the legendary Astley Cooper, who was made a baronet for removing an irritating sebaceous cyst from the head of King George IV in the middle of the night! As he did have to travel by hansom carriage from London to Brighton to do so, he deserved some recognition: but a baronetcy, surely not! Cooper was also the first person to do a vasectomy; it was on a dog.

Keats was a diligent student but found time to pursue his interest in poetry and store away the images later to be used in his poems 'Endymion' and 'Hyperion'. He shared lodgings in St Thomas's Street with two other students, for which they paid £63 a year. The premises had been found for him by none other than Astley Cooper, who seemed to take an avuncular interest in the small (Keats was 152 cm tall), rather asthenic student with a passion for verse.

At his finals in July 1816 he was examined in four subjects: translation of the Pharmacopoeia, the theory and practice of medicine, pharmaceutical chemistry and the *materia medica*. He passed with credit and entertained thoughts of becoming a surgeon. Then, like a bolt out of the blue, something crossed his consciousness which led him to abandon a promising medical career forever.

The story goes that shortly after the final exams he read George Chapman's translation of Homer's *Iliad*, and was stunned by the literary beauty of the piece. The outcome was that in October that year he wrote his first sonnet, 'On First Looking Into Chapman's Homer'. Although a newcomer in the world of letters, his sonnet was an instant success. Its rapturous reception gave him the entrée into the literary circle of Leigh Hunt, Percy Shelley, S.T. Coleridge and other literary luminaries of the time. They read it, so to speak, 'with wild surmise'. The poem is still regarded as the near-perfect example of its genre.

This success sealed the fate of John Keats. In November 1816 he turned his back on medicine to use his imaginative and innovative skills on the muse of poetry. It was to bring him everlasting fame; indeed Alfred Lord Tennyson regarded Keats as the greatest poet of the nineteenth century.

But his personal life was increasingly troubled. The poet's love affair with Fanny Brawne was going through a bad patch, and in 1818 Keats diagnosed tuberculosis within himself. His mother had died of the disease and his brother Tom was also a sufferer. In February 1820 Keats had a brisk bleeding from the lung, then another in July: ominous signs. Throughout this time he was still turning out some of his best poetic work, but his health began to go downhill, with loss of weight, night sweats and a persistent cough. Such a set of symptoms is common in this malady, especially in the polluted atmosphere of the metropolis, and as a last hope he was advised to go to Italy. He set off for Rome in September 1820.

In the Eternal City this greatest of lyric poets had further pulmonary bleeds and contemplated suicide, but was restrained, eventually dying on 23 February 1821 in his house at the foot of Rome's Spanish Steps. He was aged 25. The dwelling is now known as the Keats–Shelley House and is a place of literary pilgrimage.

William Somerset Maugham (1874–1965)

In October 1897, another of the medical profession's most famous sons qualified at St Thomas's Medical School in London, one of England's greatest training schools for doctors. He was offered a job in obstetrics, but turned it down to pursue the much more chancy calling of being a full-time writer, and it is in this field—mainly as a master short-story writer—where William Somerset Maugham gained his fame.

Of Irish origins, Maugham was born in 1874 in Paris, where his father was the legal adviser to the British Embassy. He was the youngest son. Like Keats, he was orphaned at a young age: when he was eight his mother died in childbirth, and when he was ten his father died of stomach cancer, whereupon Maugham was shunted off to live with an uncle and attend King's School in Canterbury. In his final year at school he realised he wanted to be a writer, a vocation of perceived disrepute that was quite alien to his uncle's conservative thinking. The boy's second choice was the law, but with three brothers who were lawyers, he thought enough was enough, so he cast about for another profession to follow. Initially he read philosophy and literature at Heidelberg University in Germany, but preferred to live in England, so left and enrolled at St Thomas's Medical School. Medicine, like the law, was regarded as a solid, stable and above all respectable way of earning a living. That was in 1892.

Maugham was afflicted by a marked stammer, was shy by nature and seems to have made little impression at medical school on either staff or students. As a result, in his student days he turned to writing, partly at least because it is a solitary occupation not involving much verbal communication. Nonetheless he had to 'walk the wards' and take medical case notes, interact with the nursing staff and the like. Later he gave a good description of the daily routine in his magnificent autobiographical novel *Of Human Bondage*, published in

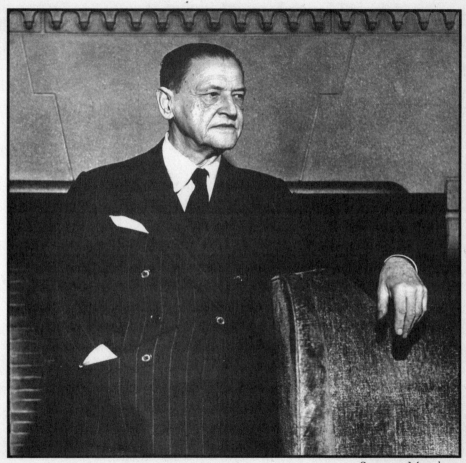

Somerset Maugham

1915 and said to have sold ten million copies. He also wrote warmly about his landlady, the splendid Mrs Freeman, in his book *Cakes and Ale*, which appeared in 1930. (Her establishment was ten minutes' walk from the hospital and she charged 18 shillings a week board and another 12 shillings for meals. When I started at medical school in Liverpool 55 years later, a week's full board had only gone up by 10 shillings.)

Dissecting cadavers held little joy for Maugham, who was more interested in visiting the live theatre to see Henry Irving and Ellen Terry tread the boards. But he did keep a notebook of events in his medical life which proved invaluable for background information later. During first year at St Thomas's he began to write plays; they were all rejected.

He proceeded to the clinical years, which he described later through the medium of Philip Carey, the medical student in *Of Human Bondage*. While doing his obstetrics in his fifth year Maugham did the required stint on the 'district'; that is, going into the London slums near the hospital and aiding in the delivery of babies at home. A midwife was always present to metaphorically hold his hand, which was just as well: Lambeth, where he worked, must have been a particularly fecund area as he managed to notch up 63 deliveries in around three weeks, or about three a day. He would need some nearby skilled help in those circumstances, as well as a bit of stamina.

Following the death of his mother, young Maugham seemed to develop an obsession about women dying in labour, and later it became a recurring theme in his novels. Doubtless he saw a few such deaths in the challenging lower socio-economic borough of Lambeth.

During the summer of 1896 he started on the rather lurid novel *Liza of Lambeth*, which dealt with adultery and the like among the working classes. Unabashed, he had called it *A Lambeth Idyll*, but with the change of name it was accepted and published in 1897 during his final year as a student. The book was priced at three shillings and sixpence, and he was given six free copies, but no advance and no royalties on the first 750 copies. But he was on his way, never to look back and never ever to work as a doctor in the community.

In the early 1900s his attempts to have his plays accepted failed, so he settled back in Paris doubtless hoping the ambience would help his muse. This proved successful and in 1908 he had four plays running at the same time in London.

At the start of World War I in 1914 he briefly served first with a Red Cross unit in France, where his by now half-forgotten medical skills came in useful, and then as a secret agent in Geneva and later Petrograd in Russia, a job which gave him plenty of ideas for gripping stories—as seen, for instance, in his book *Ashenden*, which was published in 1928.

After the war Somerset Maugham travelled in the South Seas, and then spent two years in a Scottish sanatorium while recovering from the same disease that so fatally afflicted John Keats and his mother: tuberculosis. At the time there was no specific treatment for this chronic disease; the only recommendation, if you could afford it, was rest and plenty of time in the fresh air in a place where the climate was bracing and the air pure, such as Switzerland or the Scottish Highlands. Again the experience was a source of ideas for books.

Maugham settled in the south of France in 1928, and again became a British agent early in World War II, but had to flee the country in 1940. He was an acute observer of the human condition, especially of people's psychological make-up, a skill which he doubtless gained in his early medical student days.

Dr Somerset Maugham died in 1965, having been a prolific writer of short stories, and a successful playwright who at one time was second only to George Bernard Shaw in the number of his plays running in London. He never practised medicine after qualifying 73 years before his death. But he did graciously record in *The Summing Up*, which he wrote in 1938, 'I do not know a better training for a writer than to spend some years in the medical profession.' His sum total of years thus employed was five.

Maugham and Keats were sublime examples of men who have been lost to clinical medicine, but whose subsequent actions and words cheered and uplifted many more than would have been helped by any diagnostic expertise they may have possessed.

12

The lexicographer: Peter Roget

Roget's Thesaurus—or *Roget's Thesaurus of English Words and Phrases*, to give it its full title—has been a writer's constant companion for about 150 years. 'Thesaurus' is not your everyday word, but most people can put some kind of rambling definition to it, such as, say, a list of words with related meanings. The *Concise Oxford Dictionary* gives a more obscure definition of 'elaborate lexicon'. The word 'thesaurus' itself means 'treasury' in Greek, and 'treasury of words' fits exactly.

Most people would know little about its compiler, as this is his only well-known work. In fact, Peter Mark Roget (1779–1869) was a doctor who was born in Broad Street (now Broadwick Street), Soho, London, on 18 January 1779. He happened to be born in a house that is almost opposite the community drinking-water pump which was blamed for the outbreak of cholera in 1854, and was made famous by that other determined and driven doctor, John Snow, who—after over 80 people had died that summer—demanded that the local authorities take the handle off the pump to stop it being used. (They did, thereby stopping the epidemic.)

The son of a Swiss clergyman of Huguenot origin, young Roget became obsessed with list-making. There is a personality-disorder syndrome called

'List Obsessed', and Roget became a sufferer from the age of about eight; it was probably a coping mechanism for the compulsively driven and probably rather depressed, but very bright, young boy. We would probably label him a 'savant' nowadays.

The obsession had no effect on his intellect and he was sent to study medicine at Edinburgh University Medical School, when it was the best of its kind in Britain. He graduated in 1798 and as a young graduate published works on tuberculosis (or 'consumption' as it was then known), and on nitrous oxide, which was then being tried with dubious and risky success as an anaesthetic. Anaesthetics proper were in the future, coming into use in the late 1840s.

Sad events seemed to follow him; his father and his uncle committed suicide in his presence while he was still young.

After graduation he worked in a hospital in Bristol, and in 1804 became a physician in the Manchester Royal Infirmary. Later in life he helped to organise the founding of the new medical school there, but it only actually came into being in 1874, after his death. Today there is a plaque on the wall of the medical school which commemorates the fact that Peter Mark Roget was not only a physician and compiler of the eponymously named thesaurus, but also a co-founder of Manchester's medical school.

After leaving his job in Manchester he became a private tutor to some well-to-do students and travelled with them through Europe, settling eventually back in London in 1808, by which time he had begun compiling his catalogue of words. It was on a small scale and for his own use to improve his powers of expression, and was not published in the expanded form we know today until almost 50 years later in 1852.

An enterprising man, in 1815 Peter Mark Roget invented the log slide rule, which allowed a person to use exponential powers and roots. This formed the basis of slide rules that were common currency in schools, universities and worksites for well over a century until the age of the calculator came along. Later in life our hero attempted to construct a calculating machine; it was one of the few failures in his life.

With his inventive mind driven by obsessions and compulsions almost to the level of hypomania, he still found time to help establish the Medical and Chirurgical Society of London—which went on to become the prestigious Royal Society of Medicine—while at the same time also acting as secretary to the equally prestigious Royal Society which had been founded in 1660. He held the post from 1827 to 1848. In 1834 he became the inaugural Fullerian Professor of Physiology at the Royal Institute in London, and an original member of the Senate of London University.

He also found time to write on a variety of subjects, making several contributions to a number of the early editions of the *Encyclopaedia Britannica*. Apart from that his favourite subject was the theory of optics, including how a kaleidoscope could be improved. He also published a paper, less than snappily titled 'Expansion of an optical deception in the appearance of the spokes of a wheel when seen through vertical apertures'. In 1838 he wrote a two-volume work on phrenology, which is defined as a branch of science concerned with determination of the strength of the faculties by the shape and size of the skull overlying the part of the brain thought to be responsible for them. Reading the bumps on the skull was all the rage at that time, especially in the diagnosis of putative criminals. It has, of course, been completely discredited now. There was another paper on animal and vegetable physiology, and Roget also invented a pocket chessboard.

But his crowning glory was of course his *Roget's Thesaurus of English Words and Phrases*. It was first published in 1852 when the author was in his seventies and had long given up medicine. Between 1852 and 1869 he expanded and developed the book—it ran to 28 editions in his lifetime and has never been out of print since. During that time it has been remodelled, copied and pirated, but any revisions have not shaken the principles of the original compilation, so that by now the name of Roget is inseparable from the word 'thesaurus'.

It is categorised into about 1000 topics in an arrangement that offers a choice of words to fit any context. It is an indispensable item in the armoury of all writers.

Roget died aged 91 in 1869.

13

Prolific essayist and poet: Oliver Wendell Holmes Snr

There were two Oliver Wendell Holmeses—father and son—and it is difficult to say who was the more famous. Our main interest lies in the elder, for he was a leading figure in both American medicine and in American literature during the nineteenth century.

Just to dispose of the son, so to speak, the younger Wendell Holmes was a Justice of the Supreme Court of the United States, not a doctor, and is best remembered for the 1927 case of Buck vs Bell, which had medical overtones. It concerned the State of Virginia, which sought to have the eighteen-year-old Carrie Buck, said to have a mental age of nine, sterilised. Her mother, it was alleged, had the mental age of an eight-year-old, as indeed had her mother before her. Justice Holmes agreed that the surgical sterilisation of Carrie should proceed, famously concluding, 'Enough is enough: three generations of imbeciles is enough.'

Oliver Wendell Holmes Snr (1809–1894) exhibited great compassion during his lifetime as a doctor and displayed much common sense and wisdom in his voluminous writings.

Holmes was born in Cambridge, Massachusetts, on 29 August 1809, almost

100 years to the day after his great hero Dr Samuel Johnson was born, a coincidence in which he revelled as he counted the Englishman among those who had greatly influenced his literary life. In his time Holmes was surrounded by Boston's literary elite and was friend to all the distinguished American writers of the era—Nathaniel Hawthorne, Ralph Waldo Emerson and Harriet Beecher Stowe, all of whom contributed to the enrichment of the country's literature.

His father, Abiel Holmes, was a Calvinist minister, but Oliver steadfastly rejected his severe doctrine all his life. His mother, Sarah Wendell Holmes, was light-hearted and gracious and our hero was the fourth of her five children. Surrounded by his father's large, if rather theologically orientated, library, he developed a literary talent at a young age. By the age of thirteen Oliver was writing passable poetry, and at sixteen easily passed the entrance examination for Harvard.

There he enjoyed the social round usually associated with a university lifestyle as much as he did the study and writing poetry. By the time he left, though uncertain about his future, he continued to write verse, and in 1830 moved to Boston to study medicine at the city's medical college. In 1833 he went to Paris for more advanced training, but as all the lectures were in French he had to engage a tutor to bring him up to speed with the language. He loved the city, the language, the food and the occasional wine.

It was here he first heard the theory that post-birth uterine infection—or, to give it its proper name, puerperal fever—was in fact contagious. At the time it was a great killer of post-partum women and seemed to appear from nowhere. The possibility of it being in fact a communicable disease made an impression on the young Holmes, and his proving of the fact was later to make him famous.

In 1835 he returned home and passed his final examination to become a fully fledged doctor. He continued his literary writings, winning small prizes. He ran a small private medical practice and began to privately coach anatomy and pathology to students who wanted to cram before important tests. In 1838 he was appointed Professor of Anatomy and Physiology at Dartmouth College and began to blossom as a polished lecturer, and by 1850 was a keenly sought after-dinner speaker. His first public lecture was called 'English Versification'.

In 1840 Professor Oliver Wendell Holmes married the daughter of a judge. They were to have three children. Like his father, the eldest, the jurist, had a strong personality and set views. Later in life they clashed frequently.

By 1842 cases of puerperal fever seemed to be increasing, and the interest previously shown by Holmes in Paris was roused again. The following year he published a paper in the short-lived *New England Quarterly Journal of Medicine and Surgery*, entitled 'The Contagiousness of Puerperal Fever'. By deduction and observing practices in the hospital wards he became convinced the fever was highly contagious—and, crucially, that obstetricians, nurses and midwives were active agents in its spread. His colleagues pooh-poohed the idea, and went from patient to patient without washing their hands or taking elementary cleansing precautions when examining a patient.

Shortly afterwards, a Hungarian obstetrician noted that maternal mortality in the ward attended by students was far higher than that staffed by nurses; the former had been in the highly infected post-mortem room that the latter had not visited. This obstetrician was Ignaz Semmelweis, and although he and Holmes had no contact with each other, both made the discovery more or less concurrently. Both were disbelieved and vilified at the time, but, probably on account of larger numbers of doctors being in close proximity to each other in Europe, it is Semmelweis who gained the kudos for elucidating the condition. This is remarkable as he published his findings in 1847, whereas Holmes published his findings in the distant New World in April 1843. Mind you, despite its limited distribution, the latter paper is still regarded by some to be one of the most important American contributions to the advancement of medicine.

Louis Pasteur and his discovery that germs of various sorts were the cause of infections—and not 'miasma' or rising malodorous air from swamps and the like—did not occur until the 1880s, so neither Holmes nor Semmelweis had any idea what the basic cause of puerperal fever was; they simply undertook to prove by statistical evidence that contagion existed. Holmes made an elegant plea for the protection of child-bearing women, saying 'there is no tone deep enough for regret, and voice loud enough for warning'.

In 1846 Holmes coined the word 'anaesthesia', meaning 'insensibility to touch'. He wrote to his American colleague William T.G. Morton, the first practitioner to publicly demonstrate the use of ether anaesthetics during surgery, suggesting this is what the ground-breaking technique should be called. Holmes predicted the new term 'will be repeated by the tongues of every civilised race of mankind'. A bit pompous, I would have thought, but he was right. During his lectures he was famous for stating to each new class that 'apart from opium, wine, anaesthetic agents and a few other drugs, if the whole *materia medica*, as now used, could be sunk to the bottom of the sea, it would be all the better for mankind, and all the worse for the fishes'.

In 1847 Holmes was appointed Professor of Anatomy and Physiology at Harvard University Medical School and began delivering lectures that were popular among the medical students for the next 35 years—until in fact 1882, when he turned 73 and retired.

He also became Dean of the Medical School in 1847, serving until 1853. Soon after his appointment he seriously considered admitting a woman named Harriet Kezia Hunt to the medical school. Up to then there had been no female medical students, and therefore no women doctors existed. The idea was strongly opposed by the student body and faculty members; feeling was so high it was as though he had uttered an obscenity. Miss Hunt was asked to withdraw her application. Regrettably, she did—and incredibly, Harvard Medical School was not to admit a female student until 1945. Also in the same year an Afro-American applied for admission to the medical school. The students wrote that though they had no objection to the education of black people, they did not want one in their college! So he was asked to withdraw his application too.

Another notable incident occurred during Holmes' tenure, the details of which are written up in Chapter 31. It concerns the murder by John Webster, Professor of Chemistry, of Dr George Parkman. It was Holmes who identified the bones of Parkman and who later testified at the trial with regard to Webster's teaching and research skills in the medical school.

Holmes led a busy life as an academic, but as this is a book about doctors gaining fame outside medicine the real reason he appears here is that while filling his demanding full-time post at Harvard Medical School and testing out medical theories that emanated from his fertile mind, at the same time he was also contributing numerous witty, succinct and philosophical essays to literary journals. These essays caught the public's imagination and made his name a household word to a nationwide audience and not just a few doctors.

While lecturing on tissues and bones during the day, in the evening he spoke at the local towns of Salem or Charlestown on, for instance, 'The Love of Nature' or 'Byron and Browning'. On 8 May 1857, Holmes, Ralph Waldo Emerson and James Russell Lowell brought into being the *Atlantic Monthly*, an upmarket monthly literary magazine for the discriminating and educated reader. In the first issue a piece called 'The Autocrat of the Breakfast Table' appeared. The autocrat was Oliver Wendell Holmes and he continued to contribute to the monthly magazine, eventually getting the essays together and publishing them in book form. The publication was, understandably, entitled *The Autocrat of the Breakfast Table* (1858). It was followed later by more collections: *The Professor at the Breakfast Table* (1859), *The Poet at the Breakfast Table* (1872) and *Over the Teacups* (1891).

There were more serious works, including *Our Hundred Days in Europe* (1887) and some light verse in 'The Chambered Nautilus', regarded by many as his masterpiece, and 'The Deacon's Masterpiece' in addition to informal pieces such as the 'Mutual Admiration Society'. Holmes was a prolific writer as well as a very busy teacher and clinician.

His literary efforts gave great pleasure to many people, not least to Holmes himself. He was the first who said 'every man has at least one novel in him', and was stimulated to go on and write three.

In an 1889 medical journal, the great teacher and physician Sir William Osler speculated as to whether the then 80-year-old Holmes would prefer to be remembered for his research papers on puerperal fever or for 'The Chambered Nautilus'. In a letter of reply, Holmes wrote:

My papers only come up at long intervals, the poem repeats itself in my memory . . . in writing the poem I am filled with better feelings, mental exaltation and crystalline clairvoyance. There is some selfish pleasure to be had out of the poem—perhaps a nobler satisfaction from the life-saving labour.

Some quotes from his 'Autocrat' series that have lived on include:

'Man has his will, but woman has her way.'

'The axis of the earth sticks out visibly through the centre of each and every town or city.'

'It is the province of knowledge to speak and it is the privilege of wisdom to listen.'

'Depart,—be off—exceed,—evade,—erump!'

Holmes retired from Harvard Medical School in 1882 and was made a professor emeritus. But he continued to write and travel to Europe, where he met such literary giants as Alfred Lord Tennyson and Henry James. He was awarded honorary doctorates at Cambridge, Oxford and Edinburgh, and in Paris met chemist, microbiologist and discoverer of the germ theory of infection, Louis Pasteur (doubtless they had much to talk about regarding puerperal fever). On returning home he produced his travelogue, *Our Hundred Days in Europe*.

Towards the end of his life Holmes noted he had outlived most of his friends, stating, 'I feel like my own survivor.' He died on 7 October 1894, aged 85.

14

A mighty Russian composer: Alexander Borodin

Several eminent composers have flirted with the practice of medicine: Frenchman Hector Berlioz (1803–1869), Austrian Franz von Suppe (1819–1895) and, the most famous of all, the Russian Alexander Borodin (1833–1887), who became both an eminent composer and equally well-known, medically qualified physiological chemist.

To look at the lesser medical lights first, **Hector Berlioz's** father was a doctor who hoped his son would follow in his footsteps. As a child young Hector learned the flute and guitar, and though more interested in music he went along with his old man's wishes and entered Paris Medical School in 1824. He stuck it for a year, but two things put him off continuing. Firstly, he could not stand the sight of a human corpse stretched out in the dissecting room waiting to be carved up by the students. The second reason was that he frequented the Paris Opera House and was overwhelmed by the spectacle, the sounds of the orchestra and soloists and the general musical magic of the place.

So he left medical school and enrolled at the Conservatoire, despite his mother cursing him for bringing shame on the family by choosing the bohemian life of an artist, and his father cutting off his allowance. With his strongly romantic nature he was soon successful as a composer, especially operas on the grand scale. His most famous work is probably the opera *The Damnation of Faust*.

The composer **Franz von Suppe**, following pressure from his family, was also destined for a medical career, despite being more interested in music. Again he went along with his parents' wishes and attended medical school for one year. His father then died, which allowed the young man to move to Vienna among the arty set and take up music. He was successful with his songs and frothy operettas, his most famous pieces being his overtures *Light Cavalry* and *Poet and Peasant*.

On the other hand, many physicians became very proficient in music. Perhaps the most well known was the Viennese surgeon **Theodor Billroth** (1829–1894), whose pioneering surgical treatment of stomach and duodenal ulcers which bear his name are now out of fashion, but still remembered in gastroenterological circles to this day. He was appointed Professor of Surgery at the Vienna Medical School in 1867. Several photographs of him, models of his operations and some of his pathological specimens feature prominently in the world-famous Medical Museum in Vienna. Musically he became a fine pianist up to concert pitch, but chose surgery as his main field of endeavour.

Billroth was a great friend of Johannes Brahms, who dedicated several of his works to the surgeon. The story goes that Billroth once invited his composer friend to listen to an amateur orchestra of physicians. At the conclusion of the first piece Brahms stood up and rushed out saying, 'No. No. I would rather give myself to the Vienna Philharmonic Orchestra to operate on me!'

The two great men fell out later in life, but Brahms was man enough to forgive and forget and was one of Billroth's pall-bearers at his funeral in 1894.

Which brings us at last to **Alexander Borodin**, a 'proper' doctor as well as a 'proper' composer.

Borodin was born in 1833, the illegitimate son of a Russian nobleman, Prince Gedianov, and the wife of one of his servants. Prince Gedianov registered the boy as the legal son of the servant, which in effect made the boy his own serf, but he granted the nine-year-old boy his freedom shortly before his death. He also gave the mother money and a four-storey house.

Young Alexander was a bright boy and his mother was able to afford a good education for him. He developed a strong passion for music and chemistry, an odd mixture. By the time he was fourteen he had built a laboratory at his home, and also composed some light music and a concerto for flute and piano.

In 1850 he entered the St Petersburg State Medical Academy, where early on he met a man who was to greatly influence him throughout his medical life: Professor Nikolai Zinin, one of the foremost chemists of the mid-nineteenth century, whose pioneer work on aniline derivatives led to the production of

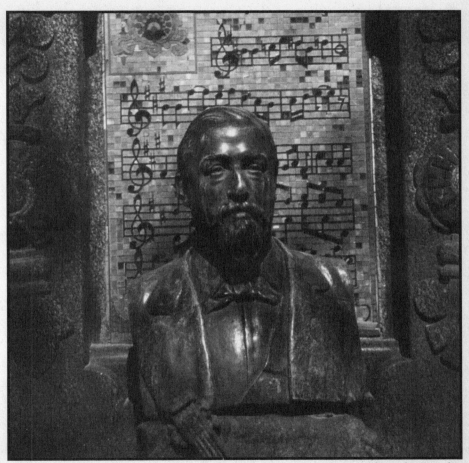

Alexander Borodin

synthetic dyes used in drugs, explosives and plastics. Alfred Nobel, of Nobel Prize fame, worked in his laboratory, and Borodin studied there as a student.

Young Borodin graduated in medicine, cum laude, in 1856, and went to work in St Petersburg Military Hospital as a junior intern. There he became a close friend of a seventeen-year-old officer in the Preobrazhensky Guards, one of Russia's most aristocratic regiments; the officer happened to be Modest Mussorgsky, who would later make his own huge contribution to Russia's nationalist musical composition.

In 1858 Borodin obtained his MD with a thesis entitled, rather obscurely, 'Analogy Between Arsenic and Phosphoric Acids'. Nevertheless Zinin, his mentor, thought the young man was spending too much time with his music rather than organic chemistry, so he sent Borodin off travelling around Europe to various chemical laboratories—one of these being that of Robert Wilhelm Bunsen, of Bunsen burner fame, in Heidelberg. It was also in Heidelberg he met a brilliant pianist and his future wife, Katerina Protopopov. She had come to that city to be treated for tuberculosis, and while there she began to spit up blood, an ominous sign. A local physician said she would not see the month out if she did not go to a warmer climate, so the two of them went to Pisa in Italy, which meant Borodin was abandoning his surgical career, at least temporarily.

They eventually moved back to St Petersburg in 1862, where Borodin was appointed Adjunct Professor of Chemistry in December that year. He married Katerina in 1863 and though they had no children and she suffered chronic bad health, they led a bohemian life and were sublimely happy, especially when Borodin became a full professor in April 1864, a post he would hold for the rest of his life. A highly regarded lecturer and research worker, Borodin, with others, was instrumental in establishing the first medical course for women in the whole of Russia in 1872.

As far as music was concerned, as well as Mussorgsky, Borodin met other like-minded artists, including the sailor Rimsky-Korsakov. They played and composed music together and soon became known as 'The Mighty Handful'. Their unifying purpose was the composition of nationalistic music—music that truly represented the feelings of the Russian people, as pioneered by Mikhail Glinka. They were opposed by another group that included Peter Tchaikovsky and Anton Rubinstein, which wanted Russian music to follow the more European pattern. Both forms were to have their place in the great corpus of Russian music.

Even with all this musical stimulus, Borodin always regarded his clinical work and teaching activities as being far more important than composing, saying: 'Composing . . . for me is only rest which takes time from my serious business as a professor . . . Men and women students are dear to me.' Fortunately he lived next door to his laboratory, so did not waste much time travelling. Even so, Rimsky-Korsakov agreed with Borodin's chief, Professor Zinin, in that he felt Alexander wasted his time on such matters as composing, rather than on his laboratory work. In his memoirs he wrote: 'He could never be in one place. Either he jumped up to see whether something was boiling over and spoiled . . . and then return to the apartment and again began to work on music', adding 'and could not accomplish his real work.'

Borodin wrote his first symphony in 1862. It was a flop due, no doubt, to his hectic life; there were too many mistakes. The second, more successful symphony came in 1872.

In 1869 the Borodins adopted a seven-year-old girl, Liza Balaneve, and later another girl, Elena Guseva. It must have inspired the composer because in the same year he began composing what was to become his most famous work, the four-act opera *Prince Igor*, based on a twelfth-century Russian saga. Naturally for Borodin it was slow progress and he appeared to abandon it in 1881; in fact it was eventually completed posthumously by Rimsky-Korsakov and Mussorgsky. Apart from opera, he did, however, compose other long pieces right up to his death in 1887.

During a trip to Germany in 1877 he met composer and pianist Franz Liszt, who was sympathetic to the Russian-biased music Borodin's group was pushing. Liszt was very impressed by Borodin's *Second Symphony* and he actively promoted Borodin's work in Germany. This brought him the international fame which has persisted to this day. The two composers corresponded and Borodin's 1880 piece *In the Steppes of Central Asia*, dedicated to Franz Liszt, cemented his fame.

Alexander Borodin died suddenly at a Military Medical Academy ball in St Petersburg on 15 February 1887. An autopsy was performed and the cause of death was established as being due to a rupture of a coronary aneurysm, leading to blood gushing into the pericardium tissue surrounding the heart to cause a fatal squeezing, or tamponade, of the heart.

In its 19 March issue of that year, the famed British medical publication, *Lancet*, wrote:

> Dr Alexander P. Borodin died suddenly probably from highly diseased coronary arteries. His [medical] published works were tolerably numerous and included a number of important articles on the estimation of nitrogen . . . In spite of his arduous professional and laboratory work, Professor Borodin found time for cultivation of the art and science of music, in which he was quite adept. He is, indeed, said to have rendered valuable service to the cause of Russian music.

With typical English lack of verve and excitement, it is rather an understated piece about a man whose life was full of emotional tension and heavy work and who gained international acclaim in his lifetime in two fields.

Katerina Borodin died a few months later of right heart failure, which could have been due to pulmonary fibrosis, consequent to her tuberculosis.

Of all medically qualified musicians Borodin was the greatest. Although he did not make a great surgeon, he expressed himself equally well in his music and medical writings. Though he once told Liszt that he was only a 'Sunday composer', Liszt neatly replied, 'Your Sunday was always a feast day', thereby summing up in one sentence the contribution that medicine's greatest musical composer had given to the muse.

15
A theatrical thespian: Sir Charles Wyndham

Published medically qualified authors are quite common, famous medical musicians are much less common, but doctors who have become professional actors are very thin on the ground. Amateur dramatics has a small coterie who enjoy acting as a form of relaxation, but full-time acting as a way of earning a living is very rare. However, there has been one outstanding exception to the rule, who trod the boards in the nineteenth century with such success that he eventually built his own theatre in London. I refer to Charles Wyndham (1837–1919), later to be knighted for his artistic endeavours.

Wyndham was born Charles Culverwell in 1837. He changed his name in 1862 when he began to act in a serious way, and has been known by this stage name ever since. Though he was born in Liverpool, his father practised as a doctor in London; Charles' own tertiary education was at Kings College, London, where he qualified as a doctor. Always interested in the stage and keen on amateur dramatics, Charles' enthusiasm was kept in check by his father, who wished to see him secure 'in a proper job'. After he duly received his Membership of the Royal College of Surgeons, however, Charles was free to follow his muse and become a serious actor.

That was at the beginning of the American Civil War in 1860 and he elected to cross the Atlantic, where, following help from the American showman P.T. Barnum, of Barnum & Bailey circus fame, he was appointed a surgeon in the Federal Army.

He was present at the battles of Fredericksburg and Gettysburg and survived under General Nathaniel Banks through the bloody Red River campaign. His army career was briefly put on hold when he made an unsuccessful appearance on the stage at New York in a company that included a certain John Wilkes Booth. Nobody was to know that Booth would obtain notoriety four years later when, as an out-of-work actor, he assassinated President Abraham Lincoln in Ford's Theatre, Washington.

Undaunted, Wyndham returned to England in 1865, where he appeared in Manchester in a play he himself had written. It was to be a turning point in his career. From then on his life was all about the theatre; he left medical practice for good. The following year he fluked an engagement at the Royalty Theatre in London playing in *Black-Eyed Susan*, and later appeared in other burlesque productions.

At that time he was an admirable and lissom dancer and, having the two skills, his career blossomed. In 1868 he was bold enough to go into management, and the following year returned to America and did an extensive tour in *The School for Scandal*. On returning to England he produced a play called *Brighton*, and although the piece is unknown now, the money he made from it was the basis of his fortune and set him on a highly successful career as a theatrical entrepreneur.

In December 1875 he took over the Criterion Theatre in London as actor/manager and stayed in the job until 1899. The Criterion was the home of farce, but it is said that Wyndham's 'vivacity and lightness of touch relieved liveliness of offence'. His business partner, leading lady and eventual wife, Mary Moore, was part of the company. If he was running short of ideas, his stand-by play was *David Garrick*, with himself as the principal character. Versatile man that he was, he translated the now-unknown play into German to take on tour, playing before royalty as well the enthusiastic hoi polloi.

By now Charles Wyndham was playing roles of middle-aged, self-controlled, cultured and charming men; with his easy, laid-back style it suited him admirably, and his large public following lapped it up.

In 1899 he built and opened his own theatre in Charing Cross Road. Without false modesty, he called it Wyndham's Theatre, and with its three-tiered, 759-seat arrangement and Louis XVI decor, it remains a well-known feature of the West End theatre-land to this day. The first play to be presented was Charles Wyndham's old favourite, *David Garrick*.

In 1903, he constructed another theatre on land he owned at the rear of his theatre in St Martins Lane. Unimaginatively, he called it the New Theatre. It was his last venture, but he continued to revive old productions from time to time and gradually and reluctantly—doubtless missing the applause—passed into retirement as an accomplished and skilled manager and actor.

He was knighted in 1902 by King Edward VII for his work in the world of theatre, and died aged 81 in 1919.

Despite his father's pious hope, Sir Charles Wyndham made little mark on medicine, but gave pleasure to thousands through his art.

16

The nearly doctor: Francis Thompson

I am hesitant to include this man among the doctor/authors, for the simple reason that he was not a qualified doctor. He did complete the required six years of medical training, but he stumbled towards the end and subsequently failed his final examination, so was never able to doff his academic mortarboard to the Chancellor of the University of Manchester to indicate he was a fully paid-up member of the medical fraternity. But in the end, as we shall see, he became so famous as a poet that the university saw fit to erect a memorial tablet on its John Owens Building recording the fact that he had been a student there.

I refer to Francis Thompson (1859–1907), a skilled poet though somewhat tragic figure in the world of medicine and art. His work had an understandable melancholy that affected many people, not least the famed 2005 Nobel Prize for Literature winner and playwright, Harold Pinter. Both Thompson and Pinter had an interest in cricket, and the influence of one on the other is dramatically illustrated by the odd fact that, as the president of the actors and writers Gaieties Cricket Club in London, at the annual end-of-season dinner every year Harold Pinter recited Francis Thompson's rather melancholic poem 'At Lord's', which talks of the 'field being full of shades', 'looking through my tears on a soundless-clapping host', and the like.

Mind you, Pinter was a well-known cricket tragic and once said he preferred cricket to sex, though hastily adding 'although sex isn't bad either'.

But let us hurry back to Francis Thompson and see, though unqualified, why he is worthy of inclusion here.

Thompson was born in December 1859 in the Lancashire cotton-spinning town of Preston where, at the time, his father, Charles Thompson, was a local general medical practitioner. In 1864 the family moved to Ashton-under-Lyne just outside Manchester, another industrial town where his father took another job as a local doctor.

At the age of eleven Francis was sent away to board at St Cuthbert's College in County Durham, north-east England. He was lonely there, but did gain recognition for his ability with the English language. He chose to follow his father into the medical profession and entered Owens College, Manchester, in 1877. It was not until a few years later that the university colleges of Manchester, Leeds and Liverpool became proper universities.

A year after entry he registered for clinical studies at the Manchester Royal Infirmary and attended the medical school for the required six years. There were three main reasons that he failed in the end to satisfy the examiners.

In 1879 he had fallen ill with an unspecified fever, and due to the conventional treatment of the day tasted for the first time the spurious delights of laudanum, also known as tincture of opium, which is opium dissolved in alcohol. At about the same time, his mother had apparently given him a copy of Thomas De Quincey's book *The Confessions of an English Opium Eater*. It fascinated him and he proceeded to fiddle with the drug, which was freely available then without prescription; his medical studies suffered accordingly.

The second reason was that he found lounging in the sun at the Old Trafford cricket ground in Manchester watching Lancashire playing their county fixtures was a much more fascinating way in which to pass the time than trampling around fusty hospital wards. At the same time he appreciated the beauty of the game, with 'the run stealers flicker to and fro', as he would put it later.

And lastly he harboured a consuming literary desire to follow the footsteps of the 'Opium Eater' in London and not study medicine at all.

Not unreasonably his father cut off the student's allowance, and Francis became even more determined to follow Thomas De Quincey's lifestyle in London. By now aged 25 he made no effort to earn a living and spent his life in the capital sleeping rough on the Embankment, and earning a pittance calling cabs for people or selling matches in Oxford Street. The rewards went on the indispensable opiate.

He never lost his literary ambition, however, and in 1887 the vagrant took a manuscript to publisher William Meynell. It contained an essay on 'Paganism Old and New' and several poems, one of which, 'Passion of Mary', was published. Some talent must have been recognised and a literary liaison developed between the two men, which grew into friendship. Knowing

Thompson's parlous state, Meynell arranged private hospital treatment and subsequent occupational therapy in the form of literary journalism.

In early February 1889 the patient relapsed and Thompson agreed to voluntarily enter the Premonstratensian Priory in Sussex, where he worked intermittently at his poems, especially 'Ode to the Setting Sun', which Meynell published later that year. After hearing and being moved by the monks singing their devotions, he wrote his most famous piece, 'The Hound of Heaven'. Published to acclaim in 1890, it reflected his own mental state, and starts:

> I fled Him down the night and down the days;
> I fled Him down the arches of the years;
> I fled Him, down the labyrinthine ways
> Of my own mind; and in the mist of tears
> I hid from Him, and under running laughter . . .

Thompson returned to meagre lodgings in London and by 1892 began again to take solace in laudanum. In December he agreed to go to the Capuchin (Franciscan) monks in North Wales to again be looked after. By June 1893 he was doing well enough to start work on a book of poetry. Later he became in demand as a storyteller and local journalist.

He returned to his publisher William Meynell, but almost at once began to take more opiates and became morose, languid and haggard. His few friends recognised that he had probably contracted pulmonary tuberculosis, which is hardly surprising in view of his lifestyle. The former senior medical student doubted this and diagnosed himself as suffering from the vitamin B deficiency beri beri. With his lifestyle it is possible, but as 'commonest things are commonest', tuberculosis was much more common and so more likely.

In November 1907 he was sent to the Hospital of St John and St Elizabeth, where the admitting registrar recorded his condition as 'morphomania'. There was some truth in this, of course, but this is more likely to have been a diagnosis of expedience: patients with tuberculosis were unwelcome as they occupied a bed for too long. The admitting doctor need not have worried: eleven days later on 13 November 1907, Francis Thompson expired. He was 48.

Addicted as he was and in the grips eventually of tuberculosis, he did visit Lord's cricket ground in London from time to time, especially if his beloved Lancashire were playing. It was about one of these Lancashire versus Middlesex games that he wrote the poem, 'At Lord's'.

Of all sports, cricket is the one with the richest literature, probably because in the early days it was the chosen game of well-educated private school and university men. With time on their hands and a literary background, they may have appreciated the contemplative pace, even tenor and subtle nuances of its stately progress. Of all that has been penned about the summer rituals of cricket, this is undoubtedly the game's greatest poem.

So it is little wonder that each year at the end-of-season dinner Harold Pinter recited the poem 'At Lord's', the last tear-jerker verse of which goes:

It is little I repair to the matches of the Southron folk,
Though the red roses crest the caps, I know.
For the field is full of shades as I near the shadowy coast,
And the ghostly batsman plays to the bowling of a ghost,
And I look through my tears on a soundless-clapping host
As the run stealers flicker to and fro,
To and fro:
O my Hornby and my Barlow long ago.

These last two named were great Lancashire players of the late nineteenth and early twentieth century, and the red rose, of course is that county's emblem.

The tablet on the wall at Manchester University dedicated to the memory of Francis Thompson, a man who never even graduated from that institution, reads:

To the Memory of
Francis Thompson, Poet,
1859–1907
Student of Owens College
1877–1884.

What so looks lovely
Is but the rainbow on life's weeping rain,
Why have we longings for immortal pain,
And all we long for mortal? Woe is me,
And all our chants but chaplet some decay,
As mine this vanishing—nay, vanished day.

17

Stand up the real Sherlock Holmes: Arthur Conan Doyle

In December 1887 there appeared in a moderately obscure British publication called *Beeton's Christmas Annual* a story by an equally obscure author. It was called 'A Study in Scarlet'. The writer sold the copyright for £25, and though he did not know it at the time, promptly missed out on making a fortune. The author was Arthur Conan Doyle (1859–1930), and as his name was appearing for the first time in print, the main character in his story was also unknown. That was soon to change.

That Sherlock Holmes became fiction's most famous detective is well known, but as this is a medically oriented essay and not a literary thesis, it is not so much Holmes himself whose life I wish to draw to your attention, but his two literary agents, so to speak, who were both medical men—the fictitious Dr Watson and the real-life Dr Conan Doyle—and, more especially, the man who by common consent is regarded as the prototype of the detective: Dr Joseph Bell, one of Conan Doyle's teachers at Edinburgh Medical School.

Just to dispose of Holmes, however, may I remind you that it is alleged somewhere in the works of his creator that he was born in 1854, became a sleuth in 1874, and retired in 1903 when he declined a knighthood. He was an expert boxer, fencer and musician, and took cocaine during periods of boredom. Allegedly he assimilated it in the form of intravenous injections of a 7 per cent solution, while at the same time indulging in indoor revolver practice! His skill was such that he could identify ash from the most obscure cigar or mud from the most distant riverbed. Indeed it was claimed that he had written a treatise entitled 'Ashes of Various Tobaccos'. By way of relaxation he is said to have played the violin and written a handbook on bee culture (not at the same time on this occasion). There seemed to be no end to his talents.

Details of Holmes' old age and death are understandably sketchy, but—and I am returning to real life now—incredibly, on the 100th anniversary of the birth of Conan Doyle in 1959, a lady called Irene Adler, purporting to be 101 years old, wrote to *The Scotsman* magazine stating that 'dear Sherlock' had died in her arms at the age of 100 after many years of keeping bees on the Sussex Downs. If true, that would have been in 1954, and is a compelling example of the whole sub-culture that has grown around the famed detective. Fiction has grown on fiction, but this imaginative fancy takes some beating.

Holmes was a somewhat antiseptic man and it would be difficult, if not sacrilegious, to actually raise a smile at his expense. But the same cannot be said of his bumbling assistant, Dr John H. Watson. Whereas Holmes was analytical and deductive, Watson was good-natured and pompous.

The story goes that John Watson was born in 1852 and studied medicine at Edinburgh. He later took the higher MD degree in London, joined the army, was posted to attend the sick in the Second Afghan War and was wounded by a 'Jezail bullet' at the battle of Maiwand in 1880. It is said he was saved from the 'murderous Ghazis' by his orderly, but contracted enteric fever and returned home convinced his health was 'irretrievably ruined'.

Lonely in London, he looked for lodgings to share and was given an introductory letter by a friend to 'a fellow who is working at a chemical laboratory up at the hospital called Sherlock Holmes'. They met in the pathology laboratory at St Bartholemew's Hospital in 1881. Holmes took one look at Watson and told him he had just returned from Afghanistan. The doctor was amazed because, of course, that is exactly where he had just come from. They were inseparable after that.

The rest is history; or rather, fiction.

After working with Holmes at the hospital, Watson settled into general practice in Paddington, but frequently visited his new best friend. Watson was a loyal companion and I suppose he represents us, the reader, being at once baffled and intrigued by the thought processes of the detective. His ingenuous artlessness adds a bit of levity to the austere Holmes, and their unlikely association lasted for over 40 years, through four long and 56 short stories, most of which appeared in the *Strand Magazine*.

If they are the fictitious characters, who were the real-life people behind them?

The creator, of course, was Sir Arthur Conan Doyle. Born in 1859, he graduated in medicine from Edinburgh in 1881 and proceeded to an MD in 1885. After two trips as a ship's surgeon he went into general practice in Southsea, near Portsmouth in southern England. There he worked with a young assistant called James Watson, and it is thought that this man at least provided the name if not the actual model for the faithful colleague of his fictitious detective.

Doyle did not attract too many patients, so he also set himself up part time just off Harley Street, the famed doctors' enclave in London, as an eye specialist. That couldn't have been too profitable either, as he published his first story in 1887, and by the time his novel *The Sign of Four* came out in 1890 he decided to abandon medicine forever and take up writing full time. From my own experience, if I'm any judge of a 'doctor-cum-writer' scenario, the patients would have thought his retirement came none too soon.

Conan Doyle did return to the profession for a short time, however, to become a civilian doctor in the Second Boer War. He was determined to do his bit and as a result was knighted in 1902—not, you will notice, for his undoubted literary skills, but for his clinical and caring efforts in that campaign. He died of a heart attack at his home in Crowborough, East Sussex, in 1930.

But by far the most interesting real-life character in the saga is the man on whom Sherlock Holmes himself is supposed to have been based. This was Conan Doyle's old lecturer in surgery at Edinburgh, Joseph Bell (1837–1911). He, it seems, was a tall, wiry man with penetrating eyes and an aquiline nose. In fact he looked rather like actor Basil Rathbone, who portrayed the detective himself in the early films of Sherlock Holmes stories.

Bell used to demonstrate a highly individualistic deductive method of diagnosis to his students where he would sit back, press his fingertips together, then fix the poor unfortunate patient with a mesmeric stare, while at the same time proceeding to note any oddities about the person.

A study of hands and fingernails revealed to Bell the nature of the man's craft; the colour of mud on the shoes the district from which he came; flakes of wood or metal on his clothing, dialect, expression, position on the chair all had their meaning to the sleuth-like doctor and had a tale to tell. Bell defined his method as 'the precise and intelligent recognition and appreciation of minor differences.' Off-putting, but effective.

A typical opening conversation by the professor has been recorded, and went like this:

'I see you served in the army.'
'Aye, Sir.'
'Not long discharged.'

'No, Sir.'

'A highland regiment.'

'Aye, Sir.'

'A non-commissioned officer?'

'Aye, Sir.'

'Stationed in Barbados.'

'Aye, Sir.'

Bell then turned to his bemused students and explained thus:

> This man was a respectful man, but did not remove his hat. They don't do that in the Army, and he would have learned civilian ways if he had been long discharged. He has an air of authority and is obviously Scottish. As to Barbados, his complaint is obviously Elephantiasis (swelling of the limbs), which is rife in the West Indies and does not occur in Britain. Anything else you want to know?

They usually didn't. They knew their place. Compare the verbatim report above of one of Bell's exposés with Sherlock Holmes' interview with a client in his short story 'The Blanched Soldier':

> 'From South Africa, sir, I perceive.'
>
> 'Yes, Sir,' he answered, with some surprise.

'Imperial Yeomanry, I fancy.'

'Exactly.'

'Middlesex Regiment.'

'That is so, Mr Holmes, you are a wizard.'

Holmes explained to his visitor:

'When a gentleman of virile appearance enters my room with such a tan upon his face as an English sun could never give, and with his handkerchief in his sleeve instead of in his pocket, it is not difficult to place him. You wear a short beard which shows you are not a regular. You have the cut of a riding man. As to Middlesex, your card has already shown me that you are a stockbroker from Throgmorton Street. What other regiment would you possibly join?'

In his obituary Bell was described as a bright and cheerful man with a spare figure and who walked head high with a jerky and energetic gait. He had, it was said, a remarkable command of the local Edinburgh vernacular, which probably means he could swear like a trooper. It was also thought at the time that the brilliant deductive skill he possessed had more to do with a preliminary glance at the case notes he had been given before appearing on the ward than any acute powers of observation. You always get knockers: I refuse to have a good story spoiled.

He occasionally made slips, and indeed tended to decry his arcane skill. It seems on one occasion he looked hard and long at a patient and without any questions asserted he was a musician. The surprised subject agreed, and Bell was at some pains to explain to the adoring students that the well-formed lips, thick cheeks and bulging eyes indicated that playing a trumpet or trombone would be his occupation. He turned to the patient and asked him which it was. The answer came straight back: 'a violin'.

Bell always asserted that his apparent 'second sight' was blindingly simple and just due to acute observation. One day a patient appeared who refused to give his name. At the end of the consultation, Bell handed the man a prescription with the full name written. He explained that he had merely read it on the visitor's hat band.

Conan Doyle was a writer whose novels have no claim to literary distinction. They are more first-class stories told in a straightforward and vigorous style than works of matchless prose. Nevertheless, he introduced a character who stimulated the founding of the Baker Street Irregulars, and a number of other societies worldwide.

But I think that Joseph Bell deserves more than a passing thought, for doubtless after one of his breathtaking acts of deduction in the outpatient department he would turn to his young assistant and say, 'Elementary, my dear Conan Doyle.'

18

Father of the short story: Anton Chekhov

Numerous medically qualified people have turned from medicine and become full-time writers, but one of the greatest of all—certainly regarded by many critics as a great playwright and the finest short-story writer of modern times—was Anton Chekhov. A master of his craft, he used his training to not only help portray many different types of doctors in his plays and stories, but also expose those hidden motives of some patients seen by doctors every day in their practice.

Anton Pavlovich Chekhov was born in January 1860 in Taganrog, a small port on the inland Sea of Azov in southern Russia. He was the third of five children; two other children had died in infancy. Of peasant stock, his grandfather, a serf, had purchased his freedom—which, paradoxically, was to create a sense of social inferiority within the family. Anton's father, a violent man who tyrannised his wife and family, had become a grocer and Anton worked in the shop as a young boy.

The business ended in bankruptcy when Anton was in his teens. The family moved to Moscow, leaving Anton and younger brother Ivan behind to continue their education at the local grammar school. With his abusive father out of the way, Anton's schoolwork improved enough for him to win at the age of nineteen a bursary worth five roubles a month for five years to study at Moscow's medical school. At that time, of the students attending Moscow State University, about 47 per cent were from noble families, most of the rest were from the Church or merchant families, and only 3 per cent had a serf background.

While studying medicine he lived once more with his family, along with two other students from his home town, and the rent they paid allowed his mother to give up her job as a laundress, and his sister, Masha, to stop working in a kitchen. Anton's father worked in a factory on the other side of the city and was seldom seen at home. The young student also helped support the family by writing innumerable comic sketches for popular 'low-brow' newspapers. This hack work allowed him to acquire the art of brevity and speed in writing, a skill he honed over time until his unrevised first draft was usually printable. He wrote under several pseudonyms, the most frequent being 'Antosha Chekhonte'. This could have been a necessary ruse as the Dean of the Medical School would have probably frowned on such frivolity by a student. But it did produce a few roubles to help support his mother.

Moscow's medical school was a good teaching institution, but not as prestigious as the Military Medical Academy in St Petersburg where, for instance, the composer **Alexander Borodin** had studied a few years previously. The fees at Moscow were five roubles per term overall, plus one rouble a week for the week's lectures. Poor students could obtain state aid, but as recompense on qualification were obliged to work without salary for three years at a major hospital. The medical course was five years, with examinations at the end of each year.

During the holidays Chekhov happily worked on the wards in a rural hospital outside Moscow helping Dr Arkhangelsky, who became a close personal friend and helped the young man professionally in later years. These working holidays were a good grounding in rural practice as he saw malnutrition, rickets, worm infestation, tuberculosis and other clinical conditions that were rife among the impoverished peasantry.

Back at the university, Chekhov was regarded as a mediocre student, but qualified without too much difficulty in June 1884. With his certificate came exclusion from poll tax and military service.

After graduation the young doctor worked briefly in the country in a hospital job, which included doing post-mortems. If a death had taken place at a distant village and he was called, the autopsy had to be done under a tree in the open air.

On top of his medical work, Chekhov continued the journalism of his student days by writing short stories and pieces for comic papers. In October of that first year out, he moved back to Moscow and set up his plate, hoping to establish a general practice in the city. He informed the local pharmacist, but it was slow going and he had to continue to write feverishly to make ends meet. The task was not made any easier by his artistic and literary friends flocking to get free treatment or paying him with vodka. An average busy general physician of the time charged five roubles and could expect to earn about 10,000 roubles a year, but Chekhov could only yearn for such largess.

In December that year he had a severe haemoptysis, or coughing up of blood from the lungs. It was his first such attack, and almost certainly due to tuberculosis, the disease which was to eventually kill him. He did not know that at the time, of course, and he wrote that painful haemorrhoids were of a more pressing concern, commenting they were 'purely the result of a sedentary life and owes something to Bacchus and Venus and heredity'. Well, possibly.

Until his tuberculosis forced a lifestyle change, between 1886 and 1897 he led a double life as a physician and writer and enjoyed both. He slowly abandoned his comic stuff and began gaining recognition in the literary world as a serious writer, his short stories being especially appreciated. His income was increasing from both disciplines and he began to seriously question whether his future lay in medicine or literature. He began to feel unfulfilled as a doctor, and suffered mild depression as a result of this inner conflict.

As early as 1888 Chekhov famously wrote to his publisher, a Mr Suvorin:

Medicine is my lawful wife and literature my mistress. When I grow weary with one, I pass the night with the other . . . neither suffer because of my infidelity. If I did not have my medical work, it would be hard to give my thought and liberty of spirit to literature.

The comment became one of his best known *bon mots*. His friend Mr Surovin, however, observed Chekhov was being unrealistic; he did not have the professional ability to work in tandem in the two fields and achieve satisfactory renown in each. Alexander Borodin alone probably had the unique ability to excel at both jobs.

Up to 1888 Chekhov was having published about a hundred humorous pieces a year, but on advice he became more thoughtful and cut down to twelve. He held that medicine had greatly influenced his literary development, saying that 'it significantly extended the area of my observations, enriched my knowledge . . . and because of my closeness to medicine, I have managed to avoid many mistakes'.

Typical of a doctor, Chekhov had an eye for the details of human behaviour, people's motives and their compromises with reality. His pages are packed with characters from all walks of life, not least among them medical men (it was scarcely yet the era of medical women). They occur in almost all his plays—except perhaps his most well known, *The Cherry Orchard*—where they seem beset with doubts, loneliness and uncertainty, lacking self-confidence and purpose, and not infrequently crossed in love. In fact, remarkably like his own life.

In 1890 Chekhov was casting about for a project to stimulate him and conceived of an investigation of conditions among residents in the notorious penal colony of Sakhalin, a narrow island off the eastern coast of Siberia.

Family, friends and especially the government discouraged the idea, but he went just the same—a trip that took him 81 days from Moscow.

Chekhov travelled all over the island interviewing the prisoners and assessing their health. Violence was rife and he found the parlous state of the children particularly distressing. He had arrived in July; by October he was exhausted and left by boat, taking the long way round via Hong Kong, Colombo and the Suez Canal to reach Odessa in early December 1890. Seeing the poverty and crush of people in the various countries along the way profoundly affected him.

In the play *Ward No. 6*, Dr Ragin is overwhelmed by running a small town hospital and withdraws into books, vodka and eating cucumbers. He is eventually committed to Ward 6 himself and has to endure the stench, beetles and mice, and patients' children sleeping in the ward. Dr Stepanovich in 'A Dreary Story' harbours love for his young ward, Katya, and cannot sleep. Dr Dorn in *The Sea Gull* is an ageing bachelor with feelings of inadequacy. Another ageing and disillusioned medic is Dr Astrov in *Uncle Vanya*, who is more interested in forestry than medicine. Most of the doctors in his plays were based on Chekhov's observations from his travels to Sakhalin and during his stint in rural practice in Russia.

All this gave a heavy and gloomy atmosphere to his work, where pessimism seems to be the hallmark. Indeed, the most frequent comment about Chekhov's plays is that nothing happens—that people just eat their dinner as they express, among ascending ennui, an inability to decide the course of their lives. Chekhov himself insisted his mature drama was comedy rather than tragedy and wished them to be produced with the lightest possible touch. He complained that Russian producers overemphasised the boredom and futility. Indeed, he insisted that *The Cherry Orchard* was 'a comedy, in places even a farce'. He seemed to make little impact for even now, a hundred years on, his craving for the light touch in presentation does not seem to have been met.

By January 1891 the writer's health had improved sufficiently following his visit to Sakhalin that he accepted a holiday as a guest of his publisher, Mr Suvorin, touring Europe during the spring and summer. He wrote up his book *Sakhalin Island* on his return, and its embarrassing revelations influenced the government to make some improvements. Chekhov hoped the book's socio-economic and medical truths would stimulate Moscow State University to accept it as a thesis and award him academic recognition with an honorary doctorate of literature. The idea was turned down without reason: perhaps he had disturbed the establishment too much.

Disillusioned by life in Moscow, Chekhov moved to a small estate at Melikhovo, about 80 kilometres from the big city. His idea was to be a local physician for nine months of the year and spend the other three months in Moscow. A medical practice can't be run like that and the move effectively ended his career as a doctor. Any medical work he did was now on an *ad hoc* basis, or as a locum.

This worked for him and the following years were among his happiest. His sister Masha settled with him and he went shooting and fishing as he wished. But by 1895 his health was deteriorating again, and his cough became very troublesome—as indeed were his haemorrhoids.

In March 1897 he suffered another severe lung haemorrhage and was admitted to a private clinic, where he was treated with subcutaneous injections of arsenic and a diet of fermented mare's milk. It seems an odd regime, and either because of it or despite it he became a semi-invalid. Whatever medical practice he was doing he now gave up entirely, and moved to Yalta in the Crimean peninsular, about 1200 km south of Moscow, to try to benefit from the drier climate. By the summer he was feeling better and went to France, staying almost eight months.

Back in Yalta, he bought a permanent home and busied himself in social work, joining a committee of doctors and wealthy residents who were building a sanatorium for the indigenous sick.

His plays were popular in Moscow, and he became financially secure, but he continued to lose weight and his cough became uncontrollable. He refused to seek medical advice; he knew the cause, but forgot the old medical saying, 'A doctor who treats himself has a fool for a doctor'.

But there was some joy at the time as he met the actress Olga Knipper, and after a turbulent courtship they were married in 1901. Their honeymoon was spent in a country sanatorium—doubtless at the sensible behest of his bride—and Chekhov was put on a strict medical regimen. The situation must have restricted their conjugal rights, to say the least. On leaving the establishment the pair seemed to act out the tortured scenarios of his plays, for she pursued her acting career in Moscow, while he sought the warmer climes of the Crimea. The newly-weds lived apart during the winter. Perhaps not surprisingly, it is then that the psychological implications of sexual involvement feature in his later stories, the most well known of which is 'Lady with a Dog'.

In 1902 Chekhov contemplated a trip to Moscow, but his doctor told Olga that any visits to the north in winter could be lethal. Chekhov was not a man to obey any instructions from his medical adviser, so he undertook the occasional trip. As there was no railway from Yalta to stations north, these illicit visits involved either a short boat trip to Sevastopol, or a six-hour coach ride to that city, to catch a train to Moscow.

Defying advice, he did journey to Moscow at the height of winter in January 1903, for the first performance of *The Cherry Orchard*, which featured his wife in the cast. It was noted by many of his old friends how thin, ill and worn he looked. The audience too were shaken by his appearance. The following January he had thoughts of going to Manchuria as a doctor to help in the Russo–Japanese war that was then raging. It was pure fantasy: he seems to have had little grasp of his parlous medical state, or was in complete denial.

With his literary powers unimpaired, in May 1904 Chekhov again went to Moscow. His loving wife promptly took him to Berlin to see a prominent chest physician, Professor Ewald. The professor's first comment was that he was amazed someone had been brought so far in such precarious health. Undeterred, Chekhov's determined spouse took her gaunt husband in June to a tuberculosis clinic in the spa town of Badenweiler in the Black Forest.

Anton and Olga were as stubborn as each other in refusing advice, for this proved to be a journey too far: the great writer-cum-doctor died there on 2 July 1904, aged 44. When his doctor wanted to apply an ice bag to his chest, the writer replied, 'One does not put ice upon an empty heart.' He then asked for a glass of champagne, drank it and died.

His body was returned to Moscow via St Petersburg in a train marked 'oysters' and he was buried there on 9 July. It could have been a scene out of one of his own works.

For much of his active adult life, our hero combined writing and general practice. He was more successful at the former, but drew most of his inspiration from the latter, managing to get into matchless prose the meaning of all those human foibles medical practitioners see every day, but the clear, concise recording of which defies most doctors' best efforts. Anton Chekhov was indeed a flower of the profession.

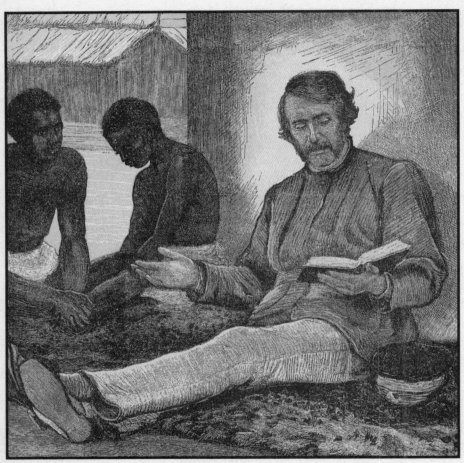

David Livingstone

PART III

Doctors who have been adventurers, inventors, athletes or politicians

19
Doctors and buccaneers

In the seventeenth century buccaneers and doctors had an uneasy, albeit a necessary, liaison. By the nature of their trade, pirates often had to call upon their medical services, however crude, and those few doctors who had seen adventure on the Spanish Main as more alluring than the daily grind in their rooms filled the bill. It was probably the closest they came to satisfying a childhood urge to run away and join a circus. Those who did take the marine alternative, however, became caught up in the cut and thrust and gore of a precarious life; but at least they did take a share of the booty.

Indeed, the word 'buccaneer' was coined by a doctor. During their heyday in the second half of the seventeenth century when pirates were plying their trade as individuals outside the law they were usually called 'privateers'. But in 1684 there appeared a book called *Buccaneers of America*, written by French surgeon/pirate **Alexandre Esquemeling (c. 1645–1707)** from Harfleur, northern France. Unlike many of his fellow so-called Brethren of the Coast, Esquemeling was articulate and well read; his book became a classic and the source of much piratical fiction. The word 'buccaneer' itself is derived from the French *boucan*, a grill for smoking dried meat on ships at sea—their common fare, I suppose. In any event, the word has passed into the language.

Before he became a surgeon, Alexandre Esquemeling had arrived on Tortuga Island near Haiti in 1666, where he worked for the French West India Company for three years. But he became footloose and bent on adventure. A lax French Government allowed the island to be a base for pirates and he elected to throw in his lot with Henry Morgan, the infamous though romanticised pirate. After three years of harsh—but doubtless lucrative—seafaring, he had had enough and either left Morgan to join a surgeon who taught him the rudiments of the craft, or returned to Amsterdam to qualify as a surgeon; history is not clear which.

Either way, Esquemeling became adept at surgery and an authority on the therapeutic worth of local plants. When he returned to his nefarious exploits he served as a surgeon during many of the exploits of Henry Morgan, and other villains. I do not suppose surgery under the skull and crossbones was very refined—almost certainly limited to cobbling together wounds and lacerations—but from the rough-and-ready experience gleaned from within his book contained a first-hand account of the piratical excesses of rape and murder. Rather incredibly, Morgan was later to successfully sue the English publishers of the tome for 'many false, scandalous and malicious reflections' on his life.

An interesting medical twist in the book concerns how the booty was divided after Morgan famously sacked Panama City in 1671. The captain himself was allotted '100 parts' of the plunder; the surgeon merely received

200 pieces of silver for the use of his medicine chest. When you consider that the 'drum-head' compensation* for injuries sustained in the course of their criminal activities included 1500 pieces of eight† or fifteen slaves for the loss of both legs, or 600 pieces or six slaves for the loss of one hand, the surgeon came cheap.

Henry Morgan (c. 1635–1688) was himself an outstanding leader, whose career pinnacle was leading 36 ships in the plunder and conquest of Panama City. It was his swan song, for shortly afterwards he 'swallowed the anchor', went straight, and retired to Jamaica where in turn he became Lieutenant Governor and a judge. He was eventually knighted by Charles II, completing a ladder of success which almost beggars belief.

Morgan led a strangely abstemious life for the rumbustious times and had enjoyed good health as a pirate. However, in 1688 in London he fell ill and was treated with dubious success by a young doctor who was to attain as great a fame in the medical profession as Morgan had in privateering. This was Sir Hans Sloane, later founder of the Chelsea Physic Garden and the British Museum, and sometime President of the prestigious Royal Society and Royal College of Physicians. Sloane Square in London is named after

---

* A drum-head compensation is the final carve-up—an idiom relating to the table used to do the distribution.

† Pieces of eight were from Spanish dollar coins worth eight *reales* which could be physically divided into eight pieces.

him; upper-class, modish young people of the area became known as 'Sloane Rangers' in the latter part of the twentieth century.

Sloane (by no means a pirate) has left us an account of Morgan's last illness when the retired ruffian was 53. He suffered from 'dropsy', due, it seems, to kidney disease, for which Sloane gave a host of treatments including poultices, clysters (or enemas) and emetics, all to no effect. A wrung-out Morgan eventually sent for another doctor, but he died just the same.

Perhaps the best-known name among the ranks of buccaneer doctors was that of **Thomas Dover (1662–1742)**, of Dover's Powder fame—a concoction that can still be found in the back room of some old pharmacies. This was a mixture of opium and ipecacuanha used as a sedative-cum-analgesic, and especially useful if diarrhoea was present. It was last recorded in the 29th edition of the pharmacists' bible, *Martindale: The Complete Drug Reference* (1989). I remember the powder well, mainly for the sweating it caused in those unfortunate enough to have it prescribed.

Dover was a successful Bristol doctor who became a medical officer on a privateering voyage on the good ship *Duke*, which circumnavigated the globe. Besides his powder, his main claim to fame was his part in the rescue of Scottish seaman Alexander Selkirk from Juan Fernandez Island off the coast of Chile on 2 February 1709. This castaway had been the navigator on the English galley *Cinque Ports*, but had quarrelled with the captain over the management of the ship. He was left marooned on an uninhabited island with his sea chest and bedding. Escape was impossible as the nearest inhabited land was 600 miles away. Selkirk was stranded there alone for 52 months, and famously became the role model for Daniel Defoe's *Robinson Crusoe*, published in 1719. After his rescue, Selkirk returned to Scotland, but never settled; he died in 1721.

Dover also popularised the use of quicksilver (mercury) for syphilis, infertility and indigestion—an odd case mix and useless in them all.

Lionel Wafer (1640–1705) was an English surgeon who joined the great Caribbean adventurer William Dampier in 1679. They raided Spanish settlements on the Central and South American coast, where Dr Wafer was severely injured following the explosion of a barrel of gunpowder. He was nursed back to health by the local Kuna Indians and was treated so kindly that in 1699 he was stimulated to write a book concerning the natural history and inhabitants of Spanish America. He also published a work about his life of pillage and looting combined with surgery, but it is the sympathetic book on the locals for which he is remembered best.

Of interest in Australia is Wafer's commander, the famous pirate William Dampier (1652–1715). Between 1678 and 1691 he was engaged in piracy off South America. During that time he diverted his course to Australia, but, having arrived, considered there was nothing worthwhile to plunder. He reformed, returned to England and in 1699 was sent by the British Admiralty to explore the antipodes in the *Roebuck*. He reached Shark Bay off the Western Australian coast and journeyed further north to name the Dampier Archipelago. The bay near Broome in Western Australia is called Roebuck Bay after the boat. Later he briefly returned to piracy, but the halcyon days of flying the Jolly Roger were over and he soon retired.

Though not a doctor, of course, Dampier was concerned about the health of his crew. He recorded that he found it very beneficial to wash morning and night, especially if suffering from the flux (diarrhoea); that old betel nuts cause giddiness but were excellent for sore gums; and that too much 'penguin fruit' produced 'heat or tickling in the fundament' (I am not sure what this means, but the mind boggles). He also became expert in the therapeutic use of many native plants.

By about 1690 various international conflicts allowed these freebooters to become legitimate privateers in the service of their respective countries. With respectability, the romantic, bloodthirsty age of buccaneers and their surgical hangers-on came to an end.

20

Napoleon's flying ambulances: Dominique-Jean Larrey

I was uncertain whether the subject of this chapter, Dr Dominique-Jean Larrey (1766–1842) was to be placed in Part I among doctors who attended to royalty and national leaders, or here as an inventor. While he was both Napoleon's personal doctor and leader of the French army medical establishment, he was also the inventor of the first ambulances made specifically for the job, so in the end I elected to put him here.

In brief, his invention was the specially constructed horse-drawn carts he devised to shift wounded soldiers from the front line to the rear, where they could be attended in comparative safety and certainly away from the stress, danger and churned-up terrain of the actual battlefield. Treatment in the rear rather than while still under fire was a new and remarkably thoughtful concept in the usual rough-and-ready army organisation of the times and saved many lives. It remains standard military practice to this day, and it was this man who transformed military medicine from a raggle-taggle outfit that frequently considered dispatching the wounded with a well-aimed bullet as the best outcome for all concerned, to something akin to a caring and, above all, a mobile operation. Perhaps it is not altogether surprising that it was Larrey who set the idea in motion, because he was famous for treating the common soldier with the same diligence and responsibility he would have the Emperor himself.

Larrey was born in the town of Beaudéan in the Pyrenees in 1766. His father died when he was a boy and he was brought up by an uncle—an army surgeon in charge of the hospital at Toulouse in southern France. It was in that city's ancient university (established in 1229) that he studied medicine. After graduation and with little hands-on experience, he entered the navy as an inexperienced student surgeon on the frigate *Vigilante*. At least he was able to study *mal de mer* and scurvy first hand, together with climate vagaries, birds and native customs in the New World, while also experiencing a near shipwreck off Newfoundland. It was a rapid learning curve.

On returning to France he entered the great teaching hospital Hôtel-Dieu in Paris (it is still there, opposite Notre Dame Cathedral), and treated some of the early trauma victims of the Revolution. In 1792 war broke out and Larrey at once joined the army. By now he was doubtless admirably fitted for such duty.

Since the invention of the cannon and other firearms in the fourteenth century, battles had become bigger and casualties began to number thousands rather than hundreds. With few exceptions—notably the armies of ancient Rome—a corp of medical officers was not found in the army before the eighteenth century. Some physicians went to serve the nobility, but the wounded rank and file looked after themselves, were tended by local inhabitants or treated by itinerant charlatans or camp followers. Logistically the wounded posed no real problem; they either tagged along with the baggage wagons as best they could, or were abandoned. In 1537 Dr Ambroise Pare witnessed an old soldier calmly cut the throats of three men who were badly wounded. The soldier then turned to Pare, saying he hoped the same would happen to him if it came to that.

Dominique-Jean Larrey showed a devotion to duty that was almost fanatical, and because of his caring attitude towards the troops he was enormously popular, though his fellow officers were not so sanguine when, on one occasion, he slaughtered some of their horses to feed his wounded men. The news of this flagrant action soon reached Napoleon, who affected displeasure and sent for the miscreant. The by-now apprehensive surgeon was asked if it was true that he had slaughtered officer's horses to feed the men. 'Yes,' replied Larrey simply. 'Well,' said the emperor, 'I will make you a Baron of the Empire.' And thereafter he was known as Baron Larrey.

Though present at many battles, Larrey was wounded on only two occasions, in Egypt and at Waterloo. He also treated Napoleon for the only injury he ever sustained—a kick on the foot from a horse. At the Battle of Aboukir Bay in Egypt he performed many amputations while under fire, and at the Battle of Borodino he personally did 200 amputations. It was these experiences which brought home to him that the best place to operate was well behind the lines, and so the germ of the idea of transporting the wounded there in what he called 'ambulances volantes' began to form.

Such ideas had been floated before, but the wagons were regarded as an unnecessary encumbrance. Queen Isabella of Spain let the wounded lie on the field of battle and then, too late, provided bedded farm wagons to transport them after the battle had passed. The Duke of Wellington during the Peninsular War thought such *folderols* (foolish nonsense) a confounded nuisance and would allow nothing to interfere with the movements of those in his army still able to stand and fight.

Similarly, at that time French regulations stated that carts to shift the living maimed should wait three miles to the rear until piggy-backed or dragged men could join them. These were huge cumbersome vehicles known as *fourgons*; incredibly, they commonly needed 40 horses or so to pull them. With the usual mud and road confusion surrounding a battle, it could take 24 to 36 hours to get to the collecting point, by which time those in need were either dead or in extremis, and if alive certainly in great discomfort. Many were left on the battlefield to be swooped on by camp followers, stripped, robbed and mutilated; friend or foe it made no difference.

Someone with medical skill, compassion and a will to stand up to military authority was needed to get some order into things. Came the crisis, came the man: Baron Larrey. This despite the fact that at the time the medical staff of the army had neither military rank nor standing, and so no military clout; they were more like civilians in uniform. But Larrey did have another very special aptitude that added weight to his forceful personality: he was a superb surgeon, a skill which was, albeit begrudgingly, recognised even by the authorities.

At the beginning of his career as he chaffed at the rear waiting for the injured, he thought he could get the wounded out on panniers slung on horses, but this proved to be impractical. The following year he pointed out to the commander, General Custine, that while the infantry had the support of mobile artillery, the same was not true for their medical needs. He sought permission to establish rapid transport on similar lines for the wounded—a flying ambulance, no less.

Custine was a 50-year-old aristocrat, Larrey was a 27-year-old provincial doctor. Normally he would have been sent packing for such a hare-brained scheme, but by significant and happy chance, when he formulated his plans in 1793 the Reign of Terror was in full cry in Paris, and the General saw it would never do for the Committee of Public Safety to learn that one of its toffee-nosed top brass had turned down a plan to help its citizens. So, amazingly, Custine gave the nod.

War being the mother of invention, Larrey rode his luck, audaciously insisting that the ambulance had to be a carriage, not cart, well sprung and light—in fact, nothing like the out dated *fourgons*. He got his wish and started at the drawing board.

Each division was equipped with twelve carriages, eight of them with two wheels for use in flat country, the others with four wheels for mountainous terrain. The back-up staff comprised 113 men, from Surgeon-Major in command, to trumpeter, who doubled as surgical instruments carrier, to drummer boy who acted as dressing carrier, to two farriers, whose only job, fortunately, was to attend the horses. At full strength the establishment had fifteen surgeons, although these included twelve under-assistants, third class, whose surgical skills were as basic as their ranking would imply.

The smaller carriage resembled an elongated cube with two small side windows and doors at each end. The floor was able to slide out over four central rollers, and was provided with a horsehair mattress and bolster. The side panels were padded for about 25 centimetres above the floor, and four metal handles were set into the floor so the planks could be pulled out and used as stretchers. At 110 centimetres wide, the base could take two patients lying full length. The whole contraption was drawn by two horses, one ridden.

The four-wheeled variety was longer and wider. The floor was fixed, but the left side opened for almost its whole length via two sliding doors, so the wounded could be lifted up and laid inside. It could accommodate four men, provided they bent their legs. A wheelbarrow was slung underneath to act as a kind of forerunner of a trolley. Power was provided by four horses, two ridden.

Thus Larrey devised one of the greatest advances ever in emergency military medicine, initiating the cardinal rule of rapid evacuation of casualties.

Larrey also provided a small but touching footnote to history when present at the Battle of Waterloo in 1815. He was actually in the French line during the final denouement, and was observed at work by the far-off mounted Duke of Wellington. When told who the man was, the Iron Duke remarked, 'Tell them not to fire on him. Give the brave fellow time to pick up his wounded.' Then, wheeling his horse, Copenhagen, the commander raised his hat in a distant greeting to the Frenchman, telling his aide, 'I salute this honour and loyalty you see yonder.' Then it was on with the slaughter.

The surgeon himself became a confidant of Napoleon Bonaparte. As well as maintaining a fine surgical dexterity until his old age, he wrote extensively on army surgery and wound treatment. In his prime and before anaesthetics, Larrey's time for removing a leg was two minutes. Doubtless at such speed, the fingers (and maybe testicles) of any slow-moving assistant were in danger of being removed in the whirl of rapid slashing.

The great surgeon eventually died in 1842, aged 76, and is still remembered as one of the most compassionate army medical officers of all time. Napoleon showed his respect in a more practical manner: he left Dr Dominique-Jean Larrey 100,000 francs in his will.

21

Two inventors of murderous contraptions: Joseph Guillotin and Richard Jordan Gatling

The two famous doctors reviewed here may not have actually murdered anyone personally but they were certainly involved in countless deaths, usually in the name of freedom or, less commonly as in our first subject, in what they saw as an act of common humanity. One of the two medical men lived in the eighteenth century, when revolution and wars were in the air. The second was a product of the second half of the nineteenth century, when the threat of war around the globe seemed to demand quick ways of killing people. The name of each is well known even today.

Dr Joseph Ignace Guillotin (1738–1814)

Most of the men and women who have achieved greatness—or maybe had greatness thrust upon them—in areas other than clinical medicine are remembered with pride and affection. Some, however, are not. In particular, history has dealt harshly with the diagnostic acumen and demonstrable kindness of Dr Joseph Guillotin. This side of his character, however, is hardly ever recounted when we morbidly recall his extramural activities during the French Revolution.

Guillotin was born on 28 May 1738 in a small town to the north of Bordeaux. In view of forthcoming events, he had what may be called a portentous start to life when he arrived prematurely, due, so the family later claimed, to his mother having been startled by the screams of a man being broken on the wheel, a particularly severe form of punishment at the time. If true, which is questionable, I am sure it is fanciful to think this influenced his life.

He trained initially as a Jesuit priest and obtained a Master of Arts from the University of Bordeaux, where he later taught literature. But he changed his objectives in life and elected to travel to Paris to study medicine. He transferred later to Rheims where he obtained a medical diploma of some kind, then returned to Paris to graduate in the customary manner in 1770.

Guillotin continued on in the academic life and taught in the Faculty of Medicine in Paris, where, as a diversion from his clinical work, he wrote reports on rabies, the medicinal use of vinegar, and swamp drainage—all commendable medical pursuits if trying to impress the Faculty. As regards his rabies research, however, being a man of the times, he concluded that convicts should be used in clinical trials, a decision at odds with his otherwise caring persona.

Later in 1784 he sat on a commission appointed by Louis XVI to investigate the dubious activities of Franz Mesmer and his hypnotic séances, or 'mesmerism' as it came to be called. The board members were a distinguished lot, including the chemist Antoine Lavoisier and the American patriot/scientist/printer Benjamin Franklin. To gain a place among this elite body was an indication of the respect in which he was held. Incidentally, the committee concluded that Mesmer was a charlatan, and his cures with 'magnetic fluid' they regarded as being due to the patients' imaginations.

In the ambient political climate, Guillotin took up the cause of the common people and in December 1788 drafted a pamphlet entitled 'Petition of the Citizens Living in Paris'. It was concerned with the proper constitution of the States General. It became a popular tract, on the strength of which Guillotin was elected a member of the National Assembly in May 1789. His contributions were directed mainly at medical reform for the masses, so he was seen as a true and compassionate follower of the common revolutionary cause. He was the Assembly's secretary from June 1789 to October 1791 and was obviously on his way up.

He also drew attention to the terrible conditions in the main Paris hospital, the Hôtel-Dieu, where people were lying in numbers of four to six in what was most likely a verminous bed. The central ward had 800 occupants who lay terrified while operations were done in the centre of the room; most procedures had about a 20 per cent mortality. Notice was eventually taken of the parlous state of the hospital and reform did occur in 1794.

Displaying his social conscience, Guillotin was also concerned with penal reform, wishing for a more humanitarian approach to the way in which the death penalty was carried out. It was in this regard that his name was to become a household word.

Such concern did not include abolition of the death penalty itself, of course, but he felt the form it took should be quick, presumably painlessly and the same for all layers of society. He concluded that these criteria would be met if 'the criminal be decapitated; this will be done solely by means of a simple mechanism . . . that beheads painlessly'. He also hoped that fewer families, and certainly fewer children, would witness the executions.

Debate took place on the issue and several experts were called upon, including Charles-Henri Sanson, the public executioner. He explained that every blow of the sword dulled the blade and, as he only had two such weapons, there were delays for sharpening, which, not unnaturally, increased the apprehension of the victim. Sometimes decapitation with the dull blade would take two or three blows to complete, and well-to-do families bribed the executioner to guarantee a quick death by giving his weapon an extra sharpening. Sanson also deplored the nervousness of the condemned who would—understandably—not hold still, and he hoped they could at least be tied down. Perhaps, he wondered, whether a mechanical method could be devised where a blade would fall by its own weight, guided by two vertical runners with the victim secured firmly in place.

In the ensuing debate, Guillotin applauded the contention on humanitarian grounds, and ghoulishly envisaged that 'The device strikes like lightning, the head flies, blood spouts, and man has ceased to live.' Though it was a dramatic and most impressive plea for what he saw as painless justice, he became forever associated with the grisly act. His name struck fear during the Terror, and he had to bear for the rest of his life the negative reputation he acquired.

It was not an instant fame, however, for at first the idea was ridiculed in song and satire and Guillotin tried to distance himself from the debate. But the famous Comte de Mirabeau, President of the Assembly, gave such ready support that 'mirabelle' was suggested as a name for the device. Following discussions and viewing sketch plans with Guillotin, Antoine Louis, the perpetual secretary of the Academy of Surgery, actually perfected the engineering layout and design of the machine, whereupon the name 'louison' or 'louisette' was suggested as its name. But 'guillotine', rhyming as it did with 'machine', and coupled with the good doctor's former popularity, proved an unstoppable combination. It was thereby adopted, ensuring the doctor's name would live on in chill remembrance. So chill, in fact, that after the great man's death his family petitioned the French Government to change the name of the apparatus to something a little more bland and less personal. The authorities refused. So instead the family did the sensible thing and changed *their* name.

Antoine Louis presented his plans on 17 March 1792. The apparatus was built in April and first used on a felon, Nicolas Jacques Pelletier, on 25 April that year. Once launched it ran hot, and quickly became the symbol of the Revolution, with 1300 heads rolling during the last six weeks.

But the public was fickle. Towards the end of the Terror, Guillotin was arrested and imprisoned on account of having received a letter from Count

Mere who, when about to be executed, commended his wife and children to the doctor's care. He was freed in 1794, whereupon he abandoned his political aspirations and turned to medical work.

Scandalised by the unsought publicity, Dr Guillotin left Paris for Arras in northern France to become the director of a military hospital. I wonder if he did so in part to help expiate the burden of responsibility he may have felt, for doubtless he knew that Arras was the home town of the guillotine's greatest exponent, Maximilien Robespierre. In any event, it was in Arras that he took an interest in vaccination, even opening a correspondence with the Englishman Edward Jenner, who invented smallpox vaccination.

Joseph Ignace Guillotin died without heirs in March 1814, having lived through the most momentous two decades in France's history. He was a kindly and clever man who almost absentmindedly lent his name to an instrument he saw as being a humane compromise in a morbid business. Regrettably, succeeding generations have misconstrued his best intentions and given him a gruesome immortality—but, right or wrong, he was complicit in many murders committed under the guise of punishment.

Dr Richard Jordan Gatling (1818–1903)

Like Dr Guillotin, Dr Richard Jordan Gatling could not be accused of actually murdering anyone himself, but his invention certainly killed many. Though

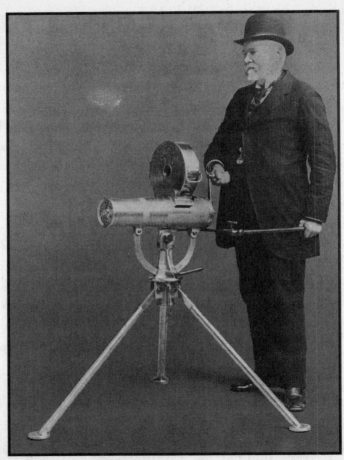

Richard Jordan Gatling

a properly qualified doctor, Gatling never practised medicine, so his story is able to be told more quickly.

He was born on 12 September 1818 in Maney's Neck, Hartford County, North Carolina, where his father was a farmer and an amateur inventor; our subject inherited the latter trait from his father. After leaving school young Gatling became a storekeeper and invented a 'wheel drill', a seed-planting device. It sold well and by 1845 he was earning enough to devote himself to selling and marketing the device, but leaving enough time to—almost as an afterthought—also go to the Ohio Medical and Dental College.

Gatling graduated as a doctor in 1850, but medicine did not hold the allure he had hoped for and he never practised the art, turning instead to business. He enjoyed the cut-and-thrust of his chosen profession and was successful with his agriculturally directed inventions. He did, though, marry a physician's daughter from Indianapolis.

During the American Civil War of the early 1860s Gatling was a supporter of the South, and he noticed that the majority of those soldiers who died did so from disease, especially typhus. Only a minority were killed by gunfire. He was later to write, in 1877:

It occurred to me that I could invent a 'machine gun' which could by its rapid fire enable one man to do as much battle duty (i.e. killing) as could a hundred acting alone, that it would to a large extent supersede the necessity of large armies, and consequently exposure to disease would be greatly diminished.

Presumably his thought was that if soldiers were to die anyway, they may as well die at once rather than linger on with debilitating illnesses.

In 1862 he founded the Gatling Gun Company to market his invention, which, rather like Dr Guillotin's invention, had in a way an element of humanitarianism. The first models were .58 calibre and had ten barrels mounted on a revolving cylinder, which was hand-cranked. In 1866 the US Government purchased the guns. The Civil War had finished by then, but the guns were used in all subsequent wars for the next 50 years until the implement was declared obsolete by the United States Army in 1911.

Following his inventive successes, Richard Jordan Gatling became more wealthy than he would have done as a medical practitioner, and anyway he preferred to use his fertile intellect to go on inventing than work out the cause of someone's illness. He patented inventions to improve toilet construction, pneumatic power and the steam-cleaning of newly clipped raw wool. But, though famous and financially comfortable, he made several unwise investments, losing several fortunes in the process.

He died on 26 February 1903 in New York.

22

Two great explorers: Mungo Park and George Bass

Mungo Park (1771–1806)

Fourshields, the farm house a few kilometres to the west of Selkirk in south-east Scotland and where in September 1771 Mungo Park was born, still stands. The name 'Mungo' is an unusual one and is from the Gaelic meaning 'amiable', a characteristic the hero of this chapter proved to have.

Mungo was the seventh of thirteen children of a well-to-do farmer. This proved to be too many to gainfully employ on the family farm, so by the time fifteen-year-old Mungo left Selkirk Grammar School he had to look elsewhere for employment. Driven, it seems, by expediency rather than altruism he became apprenticed to Thomas Anderson, a surgeon in Selkirk. After his statutory three years with Dr Anderson, in 1789 at the age of eighteen he went away to the University of Edinburgh to take the necessary diploma. Thus he qualified as a fully fledged doctor in 1791.

As he changed the course of his life only a few years later, it is not known if he was enamoured with his new profession, but after graduation he at least travelled down to London to practise his new-found art. He had a brother-in-law in the city, William Dickson—a man whose job, oddly enough, was to change Mungo Park's life. Dickson had nothing to do with the medical profession; he was a seedsman at Covent Garden. But he was also a friend of the great botanist whose name is as familiar now in Australia as it was then in the United Kingdom: Sir Joseph Banks.

Banks was a dedicated naturalist and traveller, as well as President of the prestigious Royal Society, a position he was to hold for 41 years. With such a background he was a promoter with some clout in the organisation of many expeditions at a time when journeying to distant parts of the unknown world was all the rage. He was always on the lookout for young talent, so when Dickson introduced Park to Banks he immediately asked the newly arrived jobless 21-year-old doctor if he would like to travel as an assistant surgeon on the East Indiaman *Worcester* on a voyage to Sumatra in 1792.

Well, what would you do if you were young, unattached and looking for a job? Of course Mungo Park temporarily took a break from his medical duties, signed up and sailed south to the island of Sumatra, where he collected rare plants and fish. On his return to England he wisely presented his haul to Banks and then went and took the final examinations of the Company of Surgeons. This institution became the Royal College of Surgeons shortly after, in 1800.

Again the young Dr Park was in a position to face the world and would doubtless have found being either a medical practitioner or naturalist equally congenial. In May 1794, Joseph Banks again came to his rescue and helped to make up the young man's mind by suggesting that if wanted to go to Africa it could be arranged.

The reason he could offer such a post was that he, Banks, and several influential friends ran the so-called 'African Association', whose *raison d'être* was to find out what the completely unknown and unmapped area of Central Africa was like. Mind you, the pay-off was not just to satisfy idle curiosity, but to examine the possibility of trade. The syndicate had to constantly interview candidates as, unfortunately, many starry-eyed and eager men who had gone out had died or vanished without trace and needed to be replaced. So they interviewed the young, adventurous and financially desperate Dr Mungo Park who saw African exploration as a solution to his problems, while at the same time satisfying his quest for adventure.

That was in 1794, when the Association's most pressing need was to follow up the work of Irishman Daniel Houghton, who in 1790 had been sent out to trace the course of the Niger River in West Africa, and who had got as far as sending a message back that it flowed east, whereupon he had disappeared forever. Though it was not a propitious omen, Mungo Park saw the prospect of fame as an explorer and the plaudits of his fellows very appealing and snapped up the opportunity.

The object of his task was to find out this: as the Niger flows from the west into the interior of the country, could it transport goods there? The scheme hinged on the local inhabitants being willing to trade—would they?

So on 22 May 1795 the young doctor sailed from Portsmouth in the brig *Endeavour* to Pisania, 320 kilometres up the River Gambia. There he spent about five months studying the local Mandingo language, as well as how best to treat the severe fever, possibly malaria, that he caught early on in his sojourn. He recovered sufficiently enough to leave on his own—apart, that is, from an ex-slave and a young black slave who was promised his freedom if he tagged along as a bearer. They had a horse and two asses, and for their defence they carried a brace of pistols and two shotguns.

Dr Park, then aged 25, was dressed in European clothes, carried an umbrella and wore a top hat, in the crown of which he stored his notes; a quite impractical sartorial trim, but an impressive sight nonetheless. The indigenous population were, naturally enough, intrigued by the bizarre-looking party, but the ubiquitous Arab slave-traders were less amused to see anyone on their recruiting patch. Park was continually being robbed, and an Arab chief kept him prisoner for four months, after having relieved him of his coat and umbrella. Eventually he made his escape and reached the Niger River at Segu, and was able to confirm Houghton's finding that at this spot the river did in fact flow east, and not west into the Atlantic, as one would have thought.

By now Park was exhausted and suffered from a fever that laid him low for seven months in Kaarta Taura. When well enough, he managed to get a lift on a trading caravan back to Pisania, thence to England, arriving on 22 December 1797, two and a half years after leaving home.

He reported to the Africa Association who at once—and in view of the surgeon's torrid time, perhaps rather insensitively—began discussions about him going to Australia, in particular New South Wales. In his parlous physical state he understandably declined, and wrote a book on his African travels instead. This was published in 1799, was an immediate success and was later translated into several languages. It established him as a famed African explorer; the £1000 in royalties came in handy too.

Park returned to Scotland, married the daughter of his old medical chief in Selkirk, and in 1801 moved to nearby Peebles to set up a medical practice. His brass plate simply read 'Mungo Park, Surgeon'; it is now in the Museum of Antiquities in Edinburgh. He became a friend of writer Sir Walter Scott, who used Park as the prototype of Gideon Gray in his novel *The Surgeon's Daughter*.

Having tasted the excitement and dangers of African exploration, when Park was offered another expedition in October 1803 by Lord Hobart from the government's Colonial Office, he accepted. The terms were generous this time and included £5000 for outfitting the expedition, 45 African soldiers, other qualified staff and two civilians of his own choice as companions. For the latter he chose his surgeon brother-in-law, David Anderson, and George Kirk from Selkirk.

Typical of government bureaucracy, by the time the team left Portsmouth only 30 soldiers also sailed. They arrived in Pisania on 19 August 1805, where they met more delays that ensured they could not set off until the rainy season. Nevertheless, the now 34-year-old Dr Mungo Park forged ahead with his plans. As could perhaps be anticipated, many of the group became sick; the army dwindled to eleven, and eventually was left behind in a native settlement. By November only four men were left, and both David Anderson and George Kirk had died. Nevertheless the determined Park pressed on and reached the Niger, where he built a small boat to proceed further.

We know all this because Park wrote a letter to the Colonial Office stating he had raised the British flag on the boat and was sailing east 'with the fixed determination to discover the termination of the Niger or perish in the attempt', presciently concluding, 'if I could not succeed in the object of my journey, I would at least die on the Niger'. This letter and his diaries were given to his accompanying Mandingo interpreter, Isaaco, and subsequently carried safely to Gambia and so home.

They were the last communications ever received from the explorer-cum-doctor. Was he intrepid, stubbornly single-minded or foolhardy? It is difficult to say, but he was certainly brave.

What we now know is that the 4180-kilometre Niger arises in the Guinea Highlands in West Africa, and, as Park reported, does indeed flow east through what is now Mali and into Nigeria, where it takes a great curve to finish up flowing south and then west to empty via a massive delta into the Atlantic Ocean. It does not flow straight across the interior of Africa to end somewhere on the east coast, as had been hoped by early explorers and entre-preneurs. Nonetheless, it is a tremendous waterway which, after the Nile and the Congo, is the third-longest river in Africa.

From stories recounted by locals it seems Park sailed down the Niger, past Timbuktu (then in the tribal area of darkest Africa, later in the French Sudan and now in Mali) on to Bussa, where the river passes through a rocky gorge and where, if he were to proceed, he had a choice: either fight the hos-tile natives, a task for which he was ill equipped, or chance the rapids. He chose the latter, was wrecked, and all the party were drowned. His body must have been recovered as there are in existence some personal objects and his identifiable belt.

That was early in 1806, and news of the disaster did not reach Britain until five years later.

Restless by nature, the daily routine of medical practice would never have suited Dr Mungo Park, however competent he may have been. He died aged 34 and is remembered still as a determined and intrepid explorer rather than a caring doctor. A large statue of him stands in High Street, Selkirk.

George Bass (1771–1803)

George Bass was born in the same year as Mungo Park and his childhood background was not dissimilar in that his father was a tenant farmer. He was born in the hamlet of Aswarby in Lincolnshire, eastern England. An intelligent boy, he attended the grammar school in the nearest large town, Boston, and on leaving entered the local hospital to 'walk the wards'. At the age of eighteen he went to London to polish up his anatomy and surgical techniques, being admitted to the Company of Surgeons in 1789.

After gaining more practical experience, Bass joined the Royal Navy as a surgeon in 1794. He boarded HMS *Reliance*, sailing for New South Wales in the company of Matthew Flinders, who was also destined to make his name as an antipodean explorer. After arriving in Sydney Cove, Bass and his young servant William Martin explored part of the coast of New South Wales together in the 'Tom Thumb', a tiny eight-foot wooden craft.

Restricted by the size of the boat, in 1797 they transferred their equipment to an open whaleboat with a crew of six and sailed to the furthest south-east point of Australia, then west to Gippsland in Victoria and on to the present-day site of Melbourne. From his observations of the rapid tide and long south-western swell at Wilson's Promontory, Bass believed that continental Australia was separated from Van Diemen's Land (now Tasmania) by a stretch of water. Up until then the continent and island were thought to be joined. In 1798 his theory was proved correct when aboard the sloop *Norfolk* he and Flinders circumnavigated Tasmania and confirmed it was an island.

When the two returned to Sydney, Flinders recommended to Governor John Hunter that the passage between the mainland and Van Diemen's Land be named Bass Strait, to which Hunter agreed.

Bass was also an enthusiastic botanist and forwarded many of his specimens from the new territories to Sir Joseph Banks, botanist, recruiting officer for adventurers and Mungo Park's mentor.

The explorer returned to England in 1800 and married Elizabeth, the sister of his old shipmate Henry Waterhouse, captain of the *Reliance*. Within three months he was off again to distant parts; he was never to see his bride again. Bass invested in some merchandise to take and sell in Port Jackson in the Australian colony, but there was already an oversupply of his products so he had difficulty disposing of his cargo. But he did get a contract from Governor King to import salt pork from Tahiti to Sydney, where such food was scarce at the time. After calling in to New Zealand to acquire axes and the like to trade in Tahiti, Bass returned to Sydney, in November 1802 with the meat and made a good profit.

By now quite comfortably off, Bass sailed south from Sydney on 5 February 1803 and was never seen again. His plan had been to return to Tahiti, then South America to buy more comestibles to bring back to Australia. He probably met an unfriendly reception in Chile, as at the time Spain reserved the transport of goods for her ships alone and was no friend of Britain. A fight of some kind may have taken place, resulting in the death of the doctor/explorer. Rather like Dr Mungo Park, the ultimate fate of Dr George Bass is unknown.

In January 1806, three years later, he was listed by the British Admiralty as officially 'lost at sea' and his wife was granted a pension from the widows' fund.

The stories of Mungo Park and George Bass are remarkably similar and took place within an almost identical time frame, though on different continents. Both are better known as explorers than doctors, both died in mysterious circumstances—and both are well remembered 200 years on.

23

'Doctor Livingstone, I presume'

We tend not to think of Dr David Livingstone (1813–1873) as an adventurer, even an explorer, but more as a missionary, and that is really the job to which he aspired. A committed Christian, it was the perceived task of converting the 'heathens' that drew him to 'Darkest Africa', and subsequently into exploration and adventure.

Although David Livingstone is most remembered for his exploration down the Zambezi River, where he 'discovered' the falls of Mosi-oa-Tunya ('the smoke that roars')—and which he immediately renamed Victoria Falls—his first and abiding love was his Christian faith, and exploring was only seriously undertaken after his first love had been satisfied.

The famous greeting 'Dr Livingstone, I presume' was reputed to have been uttered by Henry Morton Stanley, a journalist from the *New York Herald*, who, after ten months trekking from the coast of East Africa to find the supposedly lost Livingstone, eventually found the doctor/missionary on 10 November 1871 at Ujiji, the Arab slave-trading centre on Lake Tanganyika. Stanley quotes these as his first four words of greeting in Chapter 11 of his book, *How I Found Livingstone*. Whether it is actually true or not is of little consequence, for the phrase passed into folklore and common parlance.

Typical of his era, the devout Livingstone believed that the British were the most suitable race to convert the African population to the faith, and he was more fitted than most to do just that. He saw spreading The Word as his mission, and believed divine guidance would eventually lead him to his ultimate goal: the spot where Moses once bathed in the Nile. Such was his devotion to this duty that, in the hope of preaching more clearly, Livingstone had his uvula removed in Cape Town in 1852. The uvula is the small piece of tissue that hangs down at the back of the throat; I am sure, however, that the effect of its removal on his Scottish brogue must have been minimal.

As curing the indigent sick was seen to be an essential part of this ministry work, so it was that medicine became his second love.

David Livingstone was born in Blantyre in Lanarkshire, Scotland, in 1813, into a deeply religious family. To augment the family income, at the age of ten he left school to work in a cotton mill and continued to do so until he was 24. By thirteen he was working fourteen hours a day, but such was his desire to catch up with the education he had missed at school that he attended classes in the evening for another three hours. During the day he propped up his textbooks on the spinning jenny.

In his late teens, a pamphlet written by the German missionary Karl Gützlaff (who among other feats managed to translate the Bible into Chinese) kindled a desire in Livingstone to become a missionary. At twenty he joined the London Missionary Society with a view to foreign pastoral work and was told that if he were really serious, medical expertise was a highly desirable sideline. He was deadly serious, so with money from his brother, David walked the 10 kilometres from Blantyre to Glasgow to enter the Andersonian Medical College. Fees were £12 a year and his lodgings cost 30 pence a week. During the holidays he went back to work in the mill.

After two years he went to London to study theology, coupling it with clinical studies at Charing Cross Hospital. As he could not afford to pay for the London examinations, the dedicated young man returned to Glasgow to sit them there and qualified as a licentiate of the Faculty of Physicians and Surgeons of Glasgow in 1840.

He returned south and within a week was ordained a missionary in the London Missionary Society. To fulfil his missionary goal he had been attracted specifically to working in Africa by fellow Scottish missionary Robert Moffat. A fortnight after his ordination Livingstone sailed for Africa and into history. In 1844 he married Moffat's daughter, Mary, and for the next several years they worked together in Bechuanaland, since 1966 known as Botswana. At that time it was a centre of Christian ministry and an enclave of western civilisation in Africa, founded by Robert Moffat himself.

The diseases of that continent were a complete mystery. Over the years Livingstone was to make very many observations, though he never formulated them together into any great medical treatise, and in the light of his nineteenth-century medical knowledge he often drew erroneous conclusions.

For instance, while he knew malaria was the main scourge of the continent (though its relationship with the mosquito was then quite unknown), he felt that victims who kept active suffered least and advised accordingly. He also devised the 'Livingstone Pill' for the epidemic condition, which comprised resin of jalap, calomel, quinine and rhubarb. Doubtless the quinine, empirically given as it was, may have had some therapeutic effect; the purgative nature of the remaining ingredients would have at least taken the patient's mind off things.

He observed odd practices among the native culture, including putting to death a child who cut their lower incisors before the upper—unscientific nonsense he tried hard to stop. He also noted the eating of earth, mainly among slaves and pregnant women. He could not explain this, but I am sure that nowadays we would see it as a classic sign of iron deficiency, almost certainly due to poor nutrition.

Livingstone was among the first to note the effect of the blood-sucking tsetse fly on cattle, yet wrongly thought humans immune from any diseases these insects may carry. In fact they are a vector in the life cycle of various maladies, especially sleeping sickness. He also recorded that goitre, endemic in the highlands, disappeared within a few days of drinking water from Lake Tanganyika. A perceptive observation, but as the role of iodine in the condition was quite unknown to him, the connection meant nothing. (Iodine is a trace element found in the lake.)

In the countryside Livingstone soon became more popular as a doctor than a man of a strange God. However small his therapeutic armamentarium, the locals thought that, like his firearms, his medicine was magic. Indeed they were always pressing him to show them the secret of his 'gun medicine', as they called it.

In 1849 the missionary had travelled north and discovered Lake Ngami, sailing on which aided trade routes east and west. Between 1850 and 1856 he journeyed forth again and in 1851 came across the mighty Zambezi River. In 1855 Livingstone made his most well-known discovery: Victoria Falls. By the side of this tremendous and breathtaking natural water spectacle there now stands a fine statue of the man.

Livingstone then made a trip back to the British Isles, where he was met with great acclaim and published his book *Missionary Travels and Researches in South Africa*. It gained him some sponsorship from the Royal Geographical Society to further investigate the Zambezi. His talent and fearlessness for exploring unforgiving places had left its mark and the plaudits he received stimulated his desire to continue exploring the part of Africa with which he was most familiar.

In 1859 he found Lake Nyasa (now Lake Malawi) in what was then Nyasaland (and since 1964, Malawi). On all these explorations he never missed an opportunity to garner information about tribal customs.

His wife, Mary, died in 1862. Heartbroken, he returned two years later to England where he produced his second book, *The Zambezi and its Tributaries*.

Again the Royal Geographical Society asked their favourite son to return to the 'Dark Continent', mainly to settle the disputed question regarding the source of the Nile. He attempted this mission, pressing on amid innumerable hardships about which it was useless to complain, ultimately confusing the Congo with the Nile, then falling ill and being forced to return to Ujiji. It was here on 10 November 1871 that Mr Henry Stanley found Dr David Livingstone and uttered his famous words. Livingstone recovered enough for the two men to explore the northern end of Lake Tanganyika and to establish that it had no connection with the Nile.

A devoted Christian, an enthusiastic explorer and a dedicated doctor with few effective drugs at his disposal, Livingstone was finally claimed by Africa itself. Over the years he had suffered over thirty attacks of malaria, as well as many other extremely debilitating exotic tropical diseases. Never wavering from his chosen path, he saw them as being divinely inspired tests of his devotion.

It is remarkable he survived for so long, but after 33 years in Africa it was probably none of these exotica that got him. The good doctor had always been troubled by haemorrhoids, but refused surgical treatment when on leave, feeling the blood loss relieved his headaches (another false conclusion). However, by 1871 the loss was almost continuous, resulting in chronic anaemia and loss of energy. He decided to make for the coast and seek help, but as the great man made his tortured way there he inevitably became weaker and weaker. Attacked by driver ants, squelching through marshes, feverish, exsanguinated and emaciated, in the end his men had to carry their beloved 'father' by litter, a stretcher made of branches, bark and large leaves.

Even for such a hardy battler, it was all too much: on 1 May 1873 Livingstone died in Chief Chitambo's village on Lake Bangweulu (then in tribal lands, which became Northern Rhodesia in 1911 and is now called Zambia).

There then occurred a most remarkable sequence of events. Livingstone's devoted bearers opened up his body, removed the internal organs and heart and buried them. They were replaced by salt. The corpse was then exposed to the sun for 14 days to dry, after which it was bundled up in calico and strips of bark from the myonga tree. The whole was coated by tar and strung to a pole to be carried between two men, Susi and Chuma. It took until February 1874, about ten months, to reach the coast, and until April to get to England by sea.

With contraction and flexing of the legs, the package was only 1.2 metres in length when it arrived. A post-mortem was undertaken by Sir William Fergusson, President of the Royal College of Surgeons and surgeon at the time to Queen Victoria. He recorded that the face was unrecognisable, but one feature clinched the identity: the humerus bone in the left arm had an oblique disunited fracture with a false joint. Thirty years before, Livingstone had been mauled by a lion and sustained a compound fracture of the left upper arm. It became infected and never healed, and, incredibly, while on leave years before, the missionary had consulted the same William Fergusson about the unsatisfactory union of the bone. The surgeon recognised the old lesion at post-mortem.

The story of David Livingstone's selfless life and tragic death touched all strata of society. None had done more for African geography than this missionary, doctor and explorer during 30 years of service. His record inspired other explorers, drew respect from Arab traders and the worship of the local peoples. His own simple motto was 'Fear God and work hard'. His compassionate life earned him a burial in Westminster Abbey, where his epitaph runs:

> Brought by faithful hands
> Over sea and land
> Here rests
> David Livingstone,
> Missionary, Traveller and Philanthropist.

His vast medical impact does not get a mention. Nonetheless, to help enact the final rites there were present in the Abbey not only the redoubtable journalist Henry Morton Stanley, but also Susi and Chuma, who revered his spiritual and clinical dedication enough to have carried his body over 1000 kilometres, keeping the faith for over ten months.

24

The Grace family and other cricketers

> Imagine now that out of space
> Comes the deep spirit voice of Grace—
> Old W.G.—whose mighty frame
> No more shall lumber through the game.
>
> H. Farjeon

Of all athletic activities, cricket seems to have produced not only the richest literature, but maybe sport's most memorable characters as well. Indeed, its rather contemplative tenor and tortuous subtleties have attracted all types and conditions of men and women, including a few doctors with time on their hands and usually money in their pocket. Of these, surely medicine's greatest gift to cricket must be the mighty Dr William Gilbert Grace (1848–1915). The game in which he excelled in the nineteenth century was ruminative in nature, leisurely in pace and characterised by a gentlemanly behaviour completely different from that shown in today's game, as when, for instance, the fall of a wicket is celebrated as though it heralds the end of World War II.

With his bushy beard—a luxuriant adornment he wore from the age of seventeen until his death 50 years later—massive 100 kg and 188 cm frame, and impressive sporting record, in his pomp Grace was the most recognisable male in Victorian England; a mighty man in all senses of the word. Indeed, his portrait was used as the face of God in the 1975 film *Monty Python and the Holy Grail*. His voice was imitated by cast member Graham Chapman, another medical bon vivant. Grace was variously known by his cricketing companions as the Champion, the Leviathan, the Old Man or W.G.—never ever, heaven forbid, as Bill or Gill.

As we get enough commentaries of 'tickles round the corner' or 'bowling maidens over', and this is a chapter on doctors in cricket and not the subtle nuances of the game, let us first look at the Grand Old Man's place both in medicine and cricket. As you may well imagine, the story of his medical prowess is soon told, but his cricket stories are legion.

In the 1820s his father, Henry Mills Grace, went from Somerset to London to enrol in the then combined medical schools of St Thomas's and Guy's. He studied under the redoubtable Astley Cooper, a surgeon of such distinction that his manservant earned £600 a year in bribes from queue-jumpers seeking his advice. The young graduate, however, was of a different ilk, and much preferred the fine hunting country of Gloucestershire and playing cricket to pandering to the foibles of fashionable patients. So he set up his plate as a country general practitioner in Downend, a village between Bristol and Chipping Sodbury in England's beautiful and quaint West Country.

Henry prospered and married a lady who was as keen on sport as he was,

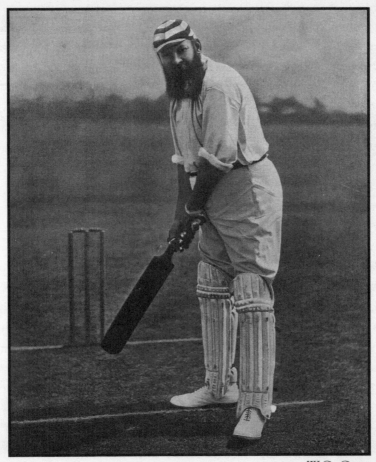

W.G. Grace

a fact that was to prove of great significance in the Grace story, as later in life she became a fastish and lethal underarm bowler who gave invaluable batting practice to her children. Of these she had nine, comprising five boys and four girls; the latter seemed to do most of the fielding to the batting of the former.

The eldest son, Henry, became apprenticed to his father in an era when you could do such things if you wanted to become a doctor. Eventually he became medical officer to the Bristol workhouse. The second son, Alfred, also qualified in medicine to finish up as the medical superintendent of the Chipping Sodbury workhouse.

The third boy, Edward, not only qualified as a doctor and became responsible for the Thornbury workhouse, but was also appointed the Coroner for West Bristol. At the age of 21 he was also regarded as the most accomplished cricketer in the west of England. During his career—when not pronouncing on death in suspicious circumstances—he managed to take ten wickets in an innings an incredible 31 times. Mind you, I should add that commonly there were then more than eleven players on each side in non-first-class fixtures and this could well have plumped up his figures. Despite that proviso, he toured Australia with George Parr's team in 1863–1864 and was known to all his cricketing mates as 'the Coroner'.

The fourth boy was the redoubtable William Gilbert, born in 1848. When his time came to follow the family tradition and study medicine, the apprenticeship system had finished, so in 1867 he entered the Bristol Medical School. It soon became apparent that he was better at cricket than fusty exams, so he changed to an establishment that he felt would be less demanding of attendance or troubled by examination results, choosing Westminster Hospital in London. Doubtless, he felt he could enter the profession by what he regarded as the back door, but alas his course was to stretch over more years than the regulations usually quoted, until in the end he finished up at St Bartholomew's Hospital to cram for his final surgery confrontation, success at which had continually eluded him.

He played cricket all during his student days, but eventually managed to fluke his exam papers. In 1879, at the unusually mature age of 31, W.G. Grace qualified as a Member of the Royal College of Surgeons of England and licentiate of the Royal College of Physicians of Edinburgh. That same year he had a batting average of 52.56 and was awarded a £1500 testimonial and two bronze ornaments for his efforts on the field. Doubtless, his examiners were forgiving supporters.

There was a last brother, George, always known as Fred, who tried to take up the profession. He was even thicker than W.G. and never did satisfy the examiners; there were limits to their forgiving nature. However, he regularly scored centuries for Gloucestershire and was regarded as one of the best rifle shots in the county. He, W.G. and E.M. (the Coroner) all played in the same England side against the Australians in 1880. Fred scored nought in each innings and died from pneumonia later that year; I cannot think the two incidents were related.

Dr W.G. Grace set up practice in Stapleton Road, Bristol, a less than salubrious area, and lived nearby in Thrissel House. He was regarded as being bluff, of jovial parts, candid in criticism and a strict disciplinarian—a set of assertive characteristics in keeping with his appearance and which had been finely honed while marshalling his men on the playing field. Nonetheless, he was popular enough in his practice to have to engage a permanent assistant, and busy enough to have to employ two locums to cover him when he went away for long periods during the summer.

As I say, unlike tell of his cricketing prowess, stories of his clinical acumen are scanty, but despite his upright, downright and forthright approach, one old lady thought well enough of him to leave him £100 and a brace of silver candlesticks in her will. He did become a public vaccinator against smallpox, and is said to have been able to smell that particular disease on entering a patient's bedroom.

His most famous medical story to come down to us occurred during the Gloucester vs Middlesex match at Clifton in 1885. W.G. batted all day for 163 not out, and then went straight from the ground to the bedside of a lady he had promised to see through her confinement. He returned the following morning to carry his bat for 221.

That much is true, but the story goes on that when asked by his team-mates how things had fared during the night, he is said to have replied, 'The child died. The mother died. But I saved the father.' For cricketers (and doctors) the truth is seldom allowed to get in the way of a good story, and almost certainly this is another example.

A well-documented incident did take place, however, in 1870 at Lord's Cricket Ground. W.G. had not qualified at this stage and was playing for the Marylebone Cricket Club against Nottinghamshire. George Summers, a Nottinghamshire player, was knocked out by a fast-rising delivery, whereupon W.G., who was fielding in his customary position near the wicket (his girth and blank refusal precluded boundary duties), went over, felt the pulse, turned to his approaching team-mates and simply remarked, 'He's not dead,' and promptly withdrew. There was some relief at this *ex cathedra*—if somewhat insensitive—statement, and the insensible Summers was carried to his hotel to take no further part in the game. He died two or three days later on the way home, presumably of a cerebral bleed consequent on a fractured skull.

There are several versions of a story that did the rounds following an incident in the 1896 Test in Sheffield, so it is probably apocryphal. Ernest Jones, the Australian fast bowler, managed to get a delivery to go right through W.G.'s splendid beard. The wicket-keeper lost sight of the ball in the hairy thicket and it went for byes. The batsman yelled down the pitch, 'What the hell do you think you are doing, Jonah?' Whereupon the abashed bowler, knowing he had committed lese-majesty of immense proportions, shamefacedly replied, 'Sorry, doctor, she slipped.'

Another unconfirmed story concerns the occasion our hero was given out caught behind the wicket first ball in a charity match. He stood his ground and shouted down the wicket for all to hear, 'They came to see me bat, not you umpire.' The hapless official knew his place and promptly called no-ball.

W.G. Grace played first-class cricket for 44 seasons, from 1864 to 1908. During that time he scored just under 55,000 runs. In his last Test in 1899, at the age of 50, he captained England against Australia. His lack of alacrity in the field was all too obvious, so he retired himself—no-one else dared do so.

He played his last first-class game in April 1908 aged 59, just four months before Don Bradman was born. It was for a splendidly named Edwardian side called the Gentlemen of England. He scored fifteen and 25. His last match ever was in a club fixture in July 1914 when, at the age of 66, he scored 69 not out in a total of 155.

This was a far cry from the occasion in 1866 when, at the age of eighteen, he scored 224 for England against Surrey and went straight from the ground to Crystal Palace to win the quarter-mile hurdle race of the National Olympian Association.

A dedicated sportsman to the end, after retirement he went on to captain the England lawn-bowls team from 1903 to 1908. I would like to see Ricky Ponting do that, or Don Bradman for that matter.

He continued his general practice in Bristol, but after twenty years he fell out with the local health authorities and moved to Kent. Knowing his personality, I am surprised it had not happened before. (During World War I German Zeppelins used to fly over his house and he would lumber outside to shake his fist and shout imprecations at them in his curious shrill, high-pitched voice—an articulation which seemed to be quite at odds with his ample stature.)

He died of a stroke on 23 October 1915 at the age of 67.

In his unique way, W.G. Grace was not only the archetypal amateur sportsman of 100 years ago, but also perhaps the most famous general practitioner of the nineteenth century. He was recognised and revered wherever he went. For instance, the train from Paddington Station, which took him back to Bristol from London, would wait if he was delayed at Lord's or the Oval. Surprisingly he was never knighted; maybe he was waiting for a peerage, say Lord Grace of Silly Mid-Off or some such.

Any kudos he extracted from life was, of course, due much more to his sporting ability than his clinical expertise, but nevertheless he was very well thought of, if not actually loved, by his patients.

He bestrode the game of cricket like a colossus, once defining his principle of cricket as 'Putting the bat against the ball', a tenet he seems to have carried through in his ordinary as well as his professional life.

Old W.G.—whose burly beard
No more is seen, no more is feared.

Some other cricketing doctors

Lead by the redoubtable W.G., the Grace brothers are the most famous family group who played cricket and carried out medical practice in a serious way. But a number of other doctors have reached the heights in that contemplative game—the 'thinking person's' ball game, if I may use that phrase. Of the approximately 3500 births and deaths of first-class cricketers who appear in the 2009 cricketer's Bible, *Wisden's Cricketers' Almanac*, as far as I can see there are only nine medical doctors (including five from one family—the Grace family, of course), plus one PhD.

This latter gentleman, incidentally, was **Dr J.A. Lester**, who died at the age of 97 in 1969. He played for Philadelphia, USA, at the beginning of the century, and was regarded by many as the best batsman America ever produced: I can hardly think there could have been much competition. He took his PhD in Education at Harvard.

The first Australian doctor to play for his country, and now long forgotten, was **Herbert Vivian Hordern**. He was born in Sydney in 1883 and was nicknamed Ranji Hordern on account of his swarthy complexion. This was a take-off of the great Indian cricketer of about Hordern's era, Prince Ranjitsinhji, the Jam Sahib of Nawanagar, whose name was shortened to Ranji in England where he played most of his cricket.

Hordern was a googly bowler and fair batsman who played seven tests before World War I. He went to Philadelphia to study medicine, and as he always considered medicine to be his primary job, his cricketing career was restricted to only 33 first-class matches, including two tests versus South Africa and five versus England. He worked as a general practitioner in Sydney and died aged 55 in 1938.

Perhaps Australia's best-known doctor-cricketer was **Dr R.H. (Reg) Bettington**, who in 1932 was also the Australian Amateur golf champion. Twelve years before this, the nineteen-year-old Bettington had gone from Kings School Parramatta to Oxford where in his first season, 1920, he created a minor sensation with his googly bowling, which mesmerised the English batsmen. Bettington went on to become the first Australian to captain Oxford at cricket, when the university team was a power in cricketing circles and ranked among the first-class county sides. He also represented Oxford at rugby and golf.

From Oxford he went to St Bartholomew's Hospital; he returned home medically qualified and became captain of New South Wales. Besides his bowling, Bettington scored five first-class centuries and once drove a ball into the press box at the Oval, the biggest ground in England.

He became an ear, nose and throat surgeon in Sydney, but met an untimely death in 1969 while on holiday in New Zealand. He was killed when his car fell 30 metres down an embankment onto a railway line.

A more recent player was **R.I. (Ric) Charlesworth**, who opened for Western Australia between 1972 and 1979 when he played 47 first-class matches for his state team. He was a somewhat leaden-footed, stodgy left-hander—characteristics quite at variance with his brilliance and fleetness of foot in the outfield, where he was a delight to watch. He writes with his right hand, but plays golf both right- and left-handedly, recording, he tells me, the same derisory score either way.

During the haemorrhage of top cricketers in the Packer era, Charlesworth was optimistically canvassed by the Perth press as an opener for the Test side. Even with the dearth of talent then available, he was, however, denied top honours by those who thought of him as more of a journeyman state player.

Such a distinction was certainly not withheld by the hockey fraternity, for Ric Charlesworth was to play hockey more times for Australia (227) than any other player. Included in that number were appearances at four Olympic games between 1972 and 1988, being captain at one of those events. He would have been at five Olympics and captained the national team twice, but Australia boycotted the 1980 Moscow Games. He was universally considered among the best two or three players in the world. Many good judges thought him to be the best of all. He retired from the game at top level after the Seoul Olympics in 1988.

From 1993 until 2000 Charlesworth was head coach of the Australian Women's hockey team, the Hockeyroos. Under his guidance they won several international trophies, including gold medals at the 1996 Atlanta and the

2000 Sydney Olympics and the World Cup in 1994 and 1998. In 2009 he was appointed coach of the Australian men's national hockey team, the Kookaburras. In that capacity he coached the team to win the World Championship in India in 2010. His tenure ends after the 2012 London Olympics.

Dr Ric Charlesworth entered federal Parliament towards the end of his playing career in 1983, after being elected the federal Member for Perth in the Lower House of Parliament, where he represented the Australian Labor Party. He resigned his seat after serving for ten years in Canberra.

His son, Jonathon Charlesworth—also a doctor, who qualified at the University of Western Australia in 2008—has recently been chosen to follow his father into the Australian national hockey team.

A name we still see from time to time in association with the management of the South African cricket team is **Dr Ali Bacher**. He played for Transvaal at the age of seventeen, and twelve times for South Africa before that country's exclusion from world sport.

The son of Lithuanian–Jewish parents, Bacher captained his country in their last series against Australia in 1969–70. In that series he led South Africa to a resounding four–nil victory. A good, if not great, participant, Bacher is best remembered in one Test match for electing to bat, after having won the toss 35 minutes before play commenced, then allowing the curator to illegally cut and mow the pitch in that half-hour. South Africa went on to score over 600 runs.

He graduated in medicine at the University of Witwatersrand, and became a general practitioner and a senior medical administrator after his cricketing days had finished.

C.B. Clarke played three tests for the West Indies in their 1939 tour of the UK. When the others returned home he stayed and enrolled at Guy's Medical School, to qualify in 1944. He was a leg-spinner whose career was ruined by World War II. However, despite his medical studies, Clarke played a tremendous amount of cricket during the war, when there were no first-class fixtures, but many morale-boosting, star-studded one-day games dotted about the country. He became a general practitioner in Pimlico, London, towards the end of the war, and after the hostilities ended he played county cricket for Northamptonshire. He later became a commentator for the BBC.

As can be seen from his wartime activities, he had intense enthusiasm as well as great natural ability. He also had a social conscience, being awarded an OBE for his community work among the West Indians in London.

One doctor who had a brief—though at times spectacular—career was **R.V. Webster**. He was yet another West Indian fast bowler and played for Warwickshire whilst studying at Birmingham Medical School. He graduated in 1964 and celebrated by returning the remarkable figures of 7 wickets for 6 runs against the mighty Yorkshire XI. He went to New Zealand and played for Otago, but medicine triumphed over sport.

The rather odd and truncated career of **Ken Cranston** is worth a mention, though he worked as a dentist, not a doctor. He qualified in Liverpool at the beginning of World War II and was considered a good club cricketer. In 1947, aged 30, he wanted to prove to himself that he could play at a higher level and gave himself two years to do so. Lancashire was looking for a captain, and appointed him, seemingly from nowhere. His accommodating father agreed to keep the dental practice going.

Cranston was so successful as an all-rounder that in his very first year he played for England against South Africa; in the Leeds Test he surprised even himself by taking 4 wickets in one over. By the time his two designated years were up, he had played eight tests, toured the West Indies and captained England. Having proved his point, Cranston, a determined personality, turning down all Lancashire's protestations to continue in the game, again took up his drills and probes and incredibly left the game forever.

The duration of a first-class cricket match precludes most doctors from taking part. I am sure many would be good enough if only they could resolve to set limits on their career, as did the single-minded Ken Cranston. Then quit while at the top.

25

Two world-beating athletes: Sir Roger Bannister and Jack Lovelock

Roger Bannister (b. 1929)

Not uncommonly, if someone is good at one thing, he or she is also good at another: it seems as though they have been favoured by the gods. One who stands out as a sportsman and academic and is a prime example of this dual blessing would be this world-class neurologist (neurology being perhaps the most intellectually difficult branch of medicine) and world-class athlete, who is still remembered by most of the population as the first man to run the four-minute mile. That was back in 1954. Later in life, in 1975, he received a knighthood, not because of his world record, nor for being an Olympic finalist in 1952—accomplishments normally sufficient for such an accolade—but for his work and dedication in the field of medicine.

Bannister was born in March 1929 in Harrow in Middlesex, England. He showed talent as a runner at school—not, let me hasten to add, at the nearby great public (private) school, Harrow, but at a local London suburban primary school. At the outbreak of World War II the Bannister family moved to a town considered to be less vulnerable to air-raid attack: Bath, in the south-west of the country.

Bannister used to practise his athleticism by running to school. He was also bright in class and resolved to study medicine when he grew up, a determination that paid off when in 1947 he won a scholarship to Oxford University to study preclinical medical subjects at Exeter and Merton Colleges. While in Oxford he pursued his athletic interest, and his times over the mile and 1500 metres began to draw attention within the sporting pages of the British press. He selflessly declined to compete in the 1948 London Olympics, preferring to concentrate on his medical studies.

In 1951 he gained the British title for the mile, and though by now engaged in demanding undergraduate clinical work of 'walking the wards' at St Mary's Hospital Medical School in London, he felt ready for the 1952 Helsinki Olympic Games. He reached the finals of the 1500 metres, but came fourth—a result attributed to the pressure of his hospital work and unorthodox training methods.

Two years later, while in his final year at St Mary's and with time for only 45 minutes training a day, he returned to the Iffley Road athletic field in Oxford, determined to break not only the world record for the mile, but to run it in under four minutes.

On 6 May 1954, being paced by his friends Chris Brasher, later an Olympic gold medallist, and Chris Chataway, later to become a cabinet minister, he achieved the unthinkable when he clocked a time of 3 minutes 59.4 seconds and passed into sporting history. Within a month the record was broken by the Australian John Landy, but it was too late: it is Bannister that athletic folklore remembers.

He never did go on to win an Olympic gold, for his selected profession took over his single-minded dedication. He retired from serious running later in 1954, graduated in medicine the same year, and published his autobiography, *First Four Minutes*, the following year at the tender age of 25.

Bannister was afraid his medical colleagues and seniors would not take his medical work seriously; running around a track might be good fun, but medicine is a tough and demanding master not given to noticing such frivolities. So when invitations came in to attend sporting events as an honoured guest, including the 1964 Olympics in Tokyo, he declined. Unlike most of the figures reviewed in this book who did medicine first and then took up another interest, it was the other way round for Dr Roger Bannister. Medicine was his new life and he was committed to it.

His special interest was neurology, which is concerned with the workings of the anatomical nervous system, rather than the psychological nervous system. In 1953, while still a student, he published two scientific papers, which were concerned with the physiology of oxygen transport through the body; his research career was on its way.

He was called up for National Service in 1958, joined the army and was posted to Aden as a medical officer. Aden is a hot and dusty place, so our hero turned his considerable mental faculties to looking at the effect of unaccustomed heat and hydration on his army colleagues. After his required two-year stint in the armed forces, he returned to London and took a job at the prestigious National Hospital in Queen Square as a Senior Resident House Physician. Despite its resounding name, the post put him among those lower ranks of the staff where all doctors start.

He continued his work on the effects of heat in various circumstances, publishing several papers on the subject, but his scholarly and methodical mind was being drawn more towards his first love, neurology. He researched the subject with terrier-like devotion, and over the years has produced more than 80 original papers focused mainly on the autonomic nervous system, which is the part of the peripheral nervous system responsible for the control of involuntary muscles like the heart, bladder and bowels—that is, organs whose bodily functions are not consciously directed.

In 1982 he wrote the first textbook on the subject and founded the British Society for Autonomic Research. He also edited several other books on related matters and received accolades from various international academic bodies, as well as being Chairman of the fledgling Sports Council of Great Britain from 1971 to 1974, and President of the International Council for Sport and Physical Recreation from 1976 to 1983. He has also served as Director of the National Hospital for Nervous Diseases as well as various athletic and medical bodies.

A modest, almost self-effacing man, Bannister's tall, thin frame and faintly academic air makes him easily recognisable at all the sporting and clinical bodies he attends. For years he continued to run mainly to maintain his own fitness, and it was during such an exercise that he was seriously injured in a road traffic accident. He recovered, but retired from private medical practice to continue his research.

Jack Lovelock (1910–1949)

A less well-known distance-runner-cum-doctor was the New Zealander John Edward Lovelock, better known to the world of athletics as Jack Lovelock, and who died in tragic circumstances a few days shy of his 40th birthday in December 1949.

He is remembered best for his part in the dramatic finish in the 1500 metres at the 1936 Berlin Olympic Games, when he won New Zealand's first-ever athletics gold medal by beating the favourite, the American Glenn Cunningham, in the world-record time of 3 minutes 47.8 seconds. The record was to stand until 1941. Before that magic moment in 1936 he also had a distinguished academic career, including a Rhodes Scholarship.

Lovelock was born in Cushington, New Zealand, on 5 January 1910 and attended the local high school, where he not only set school running records, but was dux, head boy and school boxing champion. In 1929 he went to Otago University to study medicine and in his final year became a Rhodes Scholar, taking up his prize at Exeter College in Oxford, where he resided from 1931 to 1934.

In 1932 he broke the British mile record, setting a new time of 4 minutes 12 seconds, which would have put him a long way behind Bannister in 1954. However, he competed in the 1932 Olympics and set the world record for the mile of 4 minutes 7.6 seconds in Princeton, New Jersey, the following year. Again he would have trailed Bannister.

But with all this activity away from college his academic work suffered, and he was disappointed to secure only a third-class honours degree for his BA in physiology in 1934. Rhodes Scholars are expected to obtain at least second-class honours.

In October 1934 he went to London to become a medical student at St Mary's Hospital, which was also of course the training hospital of Roger Bannister and, incidentally, the home base of Alexander Fleming, who had discovered penicillin there in 1928. While at St Mary's Lovelock competed in the Berlin Olympics, but by late 1936 the physical and financial strain of competing and attending to his hospital work was starting to tell on him, and he knew it. Further, he was suffering from knee problems that restricted his ability to set good times, a disadvantage which, as a keen competitor, he found intolerable. So he retired from running after his Olympic success, thus ensuring he left on a high note.

However, his medical problems continued, and he would inject his knee with a vaccine of dubious worth, even though concocted, it is said, by Alexander Fleming himself. Lovelock took other drugs and undertook physiological tests to try to help his knee pain. He kept a diary of these activities, but took great pains to keep his private life out of his diary. He also sustained several head injuries, mainly as a result of falling from horses. After one fall in September 1940 he was unconscious for two days. Dizziness and eyesight problems continued to affect him after this incident, and may ultimately have contributed to his early death.

Lovelock married in 1945 and two years later moved to the United States, where he took up a position at the Hospital for Special Surgery in Manhattan to work on rehabilitative medicine as an orthopaedic surgeon. A driving and fastidious personality, he was highly regarded at his job.

As a medical student at St Mary's Hospital, one of his distinguished mentors was fellow New Zealander and senior surgeon Mr Arthur (later Lord) Porritt. (A former Olympic athlete himself, Porritt became Sergeant-Surgeon to King George VI, President of the Royal College of Surgeons, and from 1967 to 1973, Governor-General of New Zealand.) In 1936, after the Berlin Olympics, Porritt made an astute observation about Lovelock, stating: 'Jack was a great worrier. He ran on nervous energy. Physically he was very fit, but mentally he was fragile, jumpy even . . . After the race in Berlin, Jack was absolutely delighted. I'd never seen him like that before and never again. He was human.'

This assessment gives us an insight into the man's personality and how and why he met his end. Being unwell from his various ailments and injuries, on top of his anxious and nervous personality, it seems that on the morning of 28 December 1949 he went to work at the hospital as usual, apparently in a normal frame of mind. But at 9.30 a.m. the secretary of his department rang his wife to say Jack was returning home. Then, while waiting at the Church Avenue subway station on Manhattan Island, he fell beneath the wheels of an approaching train and was killed instantly. He was 39 and left a wife and two daughters, the younger only a few months old.

Whether it was accidental or deliberate has been a matter of conjecture since, but he was obviously a perfectionist, and anything less than being perfect—either with his own health or in his ordinary life—could have been enough to tilt the balance. Or he simply may have had one of his dizzy turns and fallen. Once again, we shall never know.

26
Two rugby union players: Edward (Weary) Dunlop and David Kirk

Rugby union has in the fairly distant past been associated with private schools and universities, being regarded by some as a somewhat more upmarket and socially acceptable game than either its offshoot rugby league or the professional round-ball game of Association Football or soccer. Those class-distinction days are now in the past, thank goodness, but because of its university background rugby union has produced a large number of medically qualified top-class players, many of whom became internationals.

Up until about the 1950s in England, it is said that the rivalry between the various medical schools in London, each eager to win the prestigious Inter-Hospitals Cup, was so intense that, assuming they attained an absolute minimum academic standard at school, many burly and/or fleet-of-foot school rugby stars gained admission based on their value to the medical school team. The medical schools were not after a bookworm but a bruising 'rugger bugger', for success on the rugby field was where the prestige lay. If challenged on this dubious requirement for medical practice the excuse commonly given was that by playing sport the applicants were at ease socially and thus able to communicate with the patients. Very dubious, but anyway it is in the past now.

The code of football known as rugby union came as a result of a split from Association Football in 1863. A form of the game had probably been played at Rugby School in England for a couple of hundred years before this, and long before three boys at the school set down the first written rules in 1845. It is claimed that William Webb Ellis had, 'with a fine disregard of the rules of football [that is soccer] picked up the ball and ran with it'. The story is apocryphal as it first appeared in 1876 and Ellis was at Rugby School between 1816 and 1825. Be that as it may, the Rugby World Cup is now known as the Webb Ellis trophy.

Ernest Edward (Weary) Dunlop (1907–1993)

The name 'Weary' Dunlop is more associated with tremendous deeds of surgical skill under the most trying conditions in Japanese prisoner-of-war camps during World War II than rugby. He is rightly revered for his work in the forced labour camps on the notorious Thai–Burma railway where food was inadequate, beatings frequent and severe, tropical disease rampant and medical supplies almost non-existent. The compassionate Dunlop defied his captors and gave hope to the sick, placing the care of his charges before his own well-being.

That side of Weary Dunlop's life story is well known, but what may have been forgotten is that before the war and while still a medical student he was one of Australia's star rugby union players.

Ernest Edward Dunlop was born in July 1907 in Wangaratta, Victoria, where his father was a farmer. He went to school locally and when he left he became an apprentice to a local pharmacist. In 1927 he completed his pharmacy course to graduate top of his class and gold-medal winner. He elected to study medicine and went to the University of Melbourne, where as well as studying he began to play rugby.

For a sportsman he started playing quite late in life, at the age of 24. The fact that he stood 193 cm (6 feet 4 inches) tall and was fearless in his approach helped in his playing endeavours, as witnessed by the fact he progressed from the lowest-graded team to the top one very quickly. Indeed, within a year of starting the game, he was draughted into the Australian national team, the Wallabies. This is a remarkable achievement; moreover he also became the first Victorian-born player to represent the state at Test level. He made his debut against the New Zealand All Blacks in July 1932 at the Sydney Cricket Ground.

He appeared again in the first Test of 1934, when Australia beat New Zealand and went on to win the Bledisloe Cup; thus Dunlop became a member of the first Wallaby squad to have taken the cup away from New Zealand. Although his international career was relatively short on account of his medical studies, after his death in 1993 Dunlop was inducted into the Wallaby Hall of Fame—a unique honour.

Weary Dunlop graduated in medicine from Melbourne in 1934, and in

1938 journeyed to England to enrol in St Bartholomew's Medical School to study surgery. He became a Fellow of the Royal College of Surgeons later that year, which meant surgery became his first concern and his rugby-playing days were over.

Back in Australia he joined the Citizen Military Forces and later the Royal Australian Army Medical Corps, where he was commissioned as captain. At the outbreak of World War II he immediately enlisted, saying later, 'I couldn't get into the Army quick enough.'

He was posted to Java in 1942, where he was captured by the Japanese, shipped to Singapore, and then to Thailand to work as a medical officer on the infamous 'Railway of Death' which was to cost, it is said, a hundred thousand lives; Dunlop himself survived many beatings. Nevertheless, after the war he forgave the Japanese and said he had lost all hatred of the outrages they had committed.

After the war Dr Dunlop resumed his profession as a surgeon, for which he received many honours, including a knighthood in 1969 and becoming Australian of the Year in 1976. In 1988, during the 200th anniversary of the founding of the country, he was rightly named one of the '200 Greatest Australians'. In 1993 he received the unusual honour of having a Canberra suburb named after him: 'Dunlop'. His image appeared on the 1995 issue of the 50 cent coin and a bronze statue of the man stands in Melbourne's Royal Botanic Gardens.

Sir Edward (Weary) Dunlop died in early July 1993, just before his 86th birthday. He had a touch of greatness about him, and while he rightly gained national approbation for his war service, we should also remember he once played rugby union for his country.

Dr David Edward Kirk (b. 1960)

Our second medically qualified man who gained fame in rugby has also received recognition in a quite different field: the world of business.

David Edward Kirk was born in Wellington, New Zealand, but grew up in Palmerston North. He was educated at Wanganui Collegiate School and went on to Selwyn College at the University of Otago, where he graduated in medicine. While at the university he played rugby for Otago province, touring for the first time with the national All Blacks team in 1983 as a scrum-half or half-back.

He was an outstanding player: thoughtful and elusive. When the New Zealand team's tour of South Africa was cancelled on account of apartheid in 1986, he was one of just two players who refused to join a rebel team that was formed to tour in the stead of the official team. He refused on moral grounds, feeling that to go would demonstrate some sympathy with the hated South African regime.

On their return, the rebel team—appropriately named the 'Cavaliers'— were banned from playing in the next two All Black Test matches. As a result

Kirk was invited to captain the so-called 'Baby Blacks', which he did with some distinction, showing a flair for leadership on the field. When the rebels were readmitted to reform the full team he should have been demoted and the original captain, Andy Dalton, reinstated, but Dalton was injured before the match and Kirk was regarded as the obvious choice to fill his place. Kirk's confidence blossomed and he went on to lead New Zealand to victory over France in the 1987 World Cup Final, his greatest sporting moment. He played seventeen Tests for his country, eleven as captain.

To the regret of many, he abruptly retired from the game after the World Cup. He was 26. He quit to take up a Rhodes Scholarship at Worcester College, Oxford—said to be the City of Dreaming Spires and Lost Causes (unlike Cambridge, which has been scurrilously described as the City of Perspiring Dreams and Long Pauses). Medicine seemed to also have been put behind him, as Kirk elected not to expand his medical expertise but to pursue academic excellence in a quite different field: PPE—Philosophy, Politics and Economics, one of Oxford's top and more prestigious courses. It seems he had his eyes fixed on a different profession.

And so it turned out to be, for on his return to New Zealand he joined the staff of New Zealand's Prime Minister, Jim Bolger, and worked also as a management consultant. This in turn led to even higher things, for in October 2005 he became Chief Executive Officer of the large Australian company Fairfax Media, producers of the *Sydney Morning Herald*, the Melbourne *Age* and the *Australian Financial Review*. As light relief, from time to time he wrote comments on rugby when the regular journalists in his papers were not available or on strike. He left Fairfax in December 2008.

David Kirk, still going strong, seemed to have the golden touch for anything he took up. Perhaps medicine did not offer a big enough challenge, but I am sure he would have succeeded at it, just as he did at his sport and other activities.

27

Education reformist: Maria Montessori

Regrettably few women feature in this collection of doctors who have shone in fields other than medicine, but the Italian physician Dr Maria Montessori (1870–1952) is one who does. She was a first-class example of a medical professional thinking outside the square to become one of the most remarkable figures in twentieth-century education. She was also the first Italian woman to obtain a medical degree, an accolade she obtained at the University of Rome in 1894.

She was born in Chiaravalle, near Ancona in Italy, in 1870. Following graduation she at once began working with mentally defective children to become an assistant physician in a psychiatry clinic in Rome, and founding a school for 'feeble-minded' (as they were then called) children in 1899. In 1901, while treating these children, she developed a system of education for children aged between three and six years based on spontaneity of expression and freedom from restraint. She came to the conclusion that in these children the teaching approach was more important than any medication she may have ordered.

Her system of free discipline and sensory training proved so successful that children of very low intellect were able to pass the state examinations in

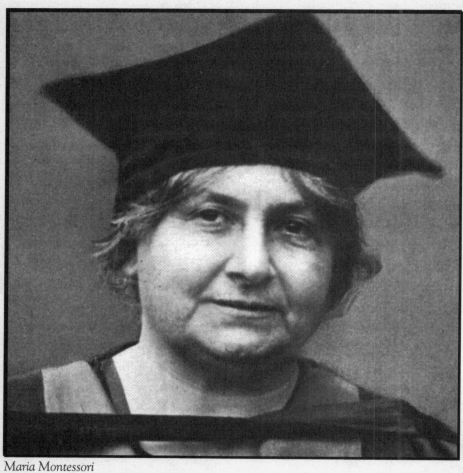

Maria Montessori

reading and writing designed for 'ordinary' children. In retrospect it has been suggested by some critics that the diagnosis of mental deficiency in the early twentieth century was unreliable, and that at least some of Dr Montessori's subjects were appreciably above borderline 'intelligence' and some of the 'normal' were below.

She was untroubled by such thoughts at the time and proceeded to apply the experience gained in 'abnormal' cases to 'normal' children, arguing that, if the mentally defective could, by educational means, be brought up to the level of normal children, still more startling results may be gained by its use on normal youngsters.

Her originality consisted chiefly in two things: first her elaborate apparatus for 'sense training', which was self-checking so that the child found out errors without correction from the teacher; and second, her contentious doctrine that the child should be free to choose his or her own activities—that they should have freedom to work at their own pace and select their own material. The teacher was to act as a supervisor or guide rather than formally lecture. This seemingly unbridled freedom grated on followers of conventional schooling: how could children know what is good for them?

Montessori adapted her methods to older children (aged six to ten) with less success, a result which gave orthodox teachers smug satisfaction. But the young doctor's main influence, however, was gained through her charm, personality, intense love of little children and her unbounding enthusiasm for both social and educational reform. She advocated individual and separate activity for each child, which was in direct contrast to the traditional custom of teaching in large classes with the pupils in rows and taught en masse.

In her first book, *The Montessori Method*, she emphasised it was better for dull or very young children to play with things of slight or no educational value than to be prematurely forced, as was usual in those days, into attempting to read and do sums with a lack of success and resulting in an antagonism to such work and a feeling of hopelessness about their own abilities.

As a result of these endeavours, Montessori was appointed lecturer in the principles, practice and profession of teaching—or, to give it the title bestowed on her in the University of Rome, Lecturer in Pedagogic Anthropology. She was charged to establish all-day schools for young children in the slum quarters of the Eternal City and opened the first Montessori School in 1907.

She published several works elaborating on her methods and travelled widely. Societies to further the cause were set up in a number of countries and training colleges were established. She received honorary degrees at several universities and in 1922 was appointed government inspector of schools in Italy.

But in October that year, Benito Mussolini's Blackshirts marched on Rome and he became dictator of the country. He and his educational establishment at first patronised the Montessori Method, but negativity supervened.

Dr Montessori appreciated the situation and left Italy in 1932. The schools she had so carefully nurtured and seen grow were banned that same year. Moreover, owing to the racial and religious tolerance fostered by their well-adjusted and tolerant founder, the principles of her teachings also fell into disfavour in Nazi Germany.

When Italy joined the German powers in the Second World War, Maria Montessori happened to be spreading the word in India, and, due to her citizenship of a now alien country, rather incredibly she and her accompanying son were interned in Kodaikanal, India, for some time as enemy aliens.

Dr Maria Montessori died in Noordwijk, Netherlands, in May 1952 while on one of her lecturing travels. She was 82.

In 1970, on the 100th anniversary of her birth, both Italy and India issued stamps to commemorate the occasion, such was the regard in which she was held.

Dr Montessori never practised medicine in the classical clinical way, but her influence in education and child psychology was wide reaching. She did not advocate complete freedom for children, once stating that: 'It is necessary to hinder . . . with absolute vigour . . . and little by little suppress all those things which we must not do.' She keenly felt her principles were 'to provide the child with work precisely adapted to his stage of development as to make much repressive discipline in the school unnecessary'.

28

Order, order: Doctors in politics

On the whole it is graduates in law who dominate the political scene of most Western countries. I suppose they are used to talking on their feet, and through their studies of the judicial process of a country have a pretty good grounding in the political system. But doctors have also had some important input into the legislative bodies of various countries and a few should be mentioned. In recent years women have come to the fore in what for centuries has been seen as the domain of men, and it is mainly women politicians I want to look at.

But first there have been some famous men.

Australia has had its fair share of medical politicians. **Sir Earle Page (1880–1961)** probably got furthest up the ladder when in 1939 he briefly became caretaker prime minister for a few weeks. He was from Grafton, New South Wales, and practised medicine before entering Parliament in 1919. He served until his death in 1961. During World War II he travelled to London as special Australian envoy to the war Cabinet.

His memoirs, published after his death, were appropriately called *Truant Surgeon*.

Doctors **Brendan Nelson** and **Bob Brown** have each been leaders of their respective political parties in Australia. Dr Brown, parliamentary leader of the Australian Greens, graduated at the University of Sydney and for some years was a general practitioner in Launceston, Tasmania, whereas Dr Nelson, former leader of the Liberal Party, graduated at Flinders University in Adelaide, and for ten years between 1985 and 1995 worked as a general practitioner in Hobart.

Looking further afield, **Dr George Clemenceau (1841–1929)** was twice the Prime Minister of France and presided over the Peace Conference in 1919. Both his father and grandfather were doctors. He studied medicine in Nantes and then Paris, where he later worked as a physician, but his republican views brought him into conflict with the government. To avoid the heat he went to the United States, working as a journalist and teacher.

On his return to France he entered the Chamber of Deputies in 1876, became leader of the extreme left and premier in 1906, and then again in 1917, acquiring the nickname 'Tiger'.

François Duvalier (1907–1971), famously known as 'Papa Doc', President of Haiti and a professed believer in Voodoo, was trained in medicine and became Director of Public Health Services of his country in 1946 and Minister for Health three years later. Following a coup, he was overwhelmingly elected president in 1957, going on to lead an autocratic and murderous regime. He was succeeded by his twenty-year-old son in 1971, who became known as 'Baby Doc', despite the fact he studied law and not medicine. Though originally appointed 'president for life', the young man was deposed in 1986.

With his smouldering good looks and reformer's passion, **Che Guevara (1928–1967)** was—and still is—a romanticised South American politician, who graduated in medicine at the University of Buenos Aires in 1953 before joining Fidel Castro's revolutionary movement in Mexico. Later he played an important part in the Cuban Revolution and held government posts under Castro. He left Cuba in 1965 to become a guerrilla leader in Bolivia, where two years later he was captured and executed.

The first President of the Republic of China was **Sun Yat-Sen (1866–1925),** a medical graduate of Hong Kong. Son of a Christian farmer, he was born near Canton (Guangzhou), but brought up by his elder brother in Hawaii. He graduated in 1892 and practised in Macao and Canton, before becoming politically active and leading an unsuccessful uprising against the Manchu in 1895. Defeated, he fled to England, only to be captured by members of the Chinese Legation in London. He managed to smuggle out a note to his former surgical tutor, Sir James Cantlie, who intervened and saved Sun Yat-Sen from almost certain death. The Chinese doctor returned to his homeland and began organising a number of failed uprisings against the rulers, to at last succeed in 1911. In February 1912 China was declared a republic, with Sun Yat-Sen its provisional president, but he resigned during the same year in favour of a military man. He died in 1925.

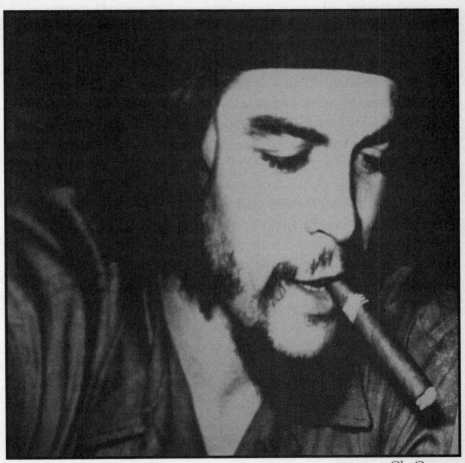

Che Guevara

In recent years Europe has produced several highly talented female medical graduates who have become influential in politics and who deserve a wider recognition than they enjoy at present.

Born in Oslo in 1939, the brilliant **Dr Gro Harlem Brundtland** became Prime Minister of Norway on three occasions, and later Director-General of the World Health Organization.

Brundtland studied medicine at the University of Oslo, graduating in 1963. She went on to Harvard to complete a Master of Public Health in 1965, whereupon she returned home and worked as a physician in the Norwegian public school health service. In 1973 she was elected to the Norwegian Parliament and in the following year became the country's Minister of Environmental Affairs.

In 1981 Brundtland was elevated to Chairperson of the Labour Party, leading her party to electoral victory the same year. As party head she became prime minister that year, serving only from February to October. But she did go on to gain the top job for two more terms between 1986 and 1989, during which time she broke with tradition by appointing eight women to serve in her eighteen-strong Cabinet.

In 1996 she retired from Norwegian politics and in 1998 took up the position of Director-General of the World Health Organization, a post she held for five years. During her term she addressed violence, which she saw as a major public health problem, and spearheaded a movement to abolish cigarette smoking. In 2004 the British *Financial Times* listed her as the fourth most influential European over the previous 25 years, after Pope John Paul II, Mikhail Gorbachev and Margaret Thatcher respectively.

In 2007 the Secretary-General of the United Nations appointed Gro Harlem Brundtland as one of its Special Envoys in Climate Change.

She married in 1960 and during all this political activity found time to rear four children. In 2002 she had an operation for uterine cancer. Brundtland now works for the PepsiCo company as a consultant and still lives in her home country.

East Germany's last head of state was **Dr Sabine Bergmann-Pohl**, who served between 5 April and 2 October 1990 and stepped down on 3 October when East and West Germany were reunited and her post became redundant.

Born on 20 April 1946 in Eisenach in the south-west of East Germany, she studied medicine at the highly regarded Humboldt University in Berlin, graduating in 1972. (Set in the ground among the cobblestones of that university's great forecourt is a tough glass window. Through it can be seen several rows of empty bookshelves: that's all. It was on that very spot where in the 1930s the Nazis burned thousands of university textbooks and manuscripts that recorded opposition to their regime. The stark simplicity of the 'empty library' memorialising this act of academic vandalism is incredibly moving.)

After graduation Dr Bergmann-Pohl specialised in lung diseases and also joined the Christian Democratic Union of the German Democratic Republic

(GDP). After winning a seat at the free elections of March 1990, she became a member of the East German legislature, or Volkskammer, and its president in April. As the GDP's Council of State had been abolished at the same time, it meant that she at once also became East Germany's head of state in what was a meteoric rise to the top job.

After the nation's reunification six months later in October, she lost her position and was named 'Minister Without Portfolio'. Between 1991 and 1998 she was Under-Secretary of State for Health within the new united Germany. She retired from politics in 2002.

Dr Michelle Bachelet was elected President of Chile in 2006 and held the post until succeeded by Sebastian Piñera in 2010. A moderate socialist politician, Dr Bachelet campaigned on increasing social benefits to help reduce the large financial gap between the rich and the poor. She also favoured free market policies for Chile and has remained popular among the electorate; after three years as president, in 2009, her approval rating was 71 per cent.

Bachelet was born in Santiago. Her mother was an archaeologist and her father an Air Force General. Following his postings, the family moved frequently, including a two-year stint in the Chilean Embassy in Washington, during which time our subject attended school and learned to speak fluent English.

Michelle Bachelet entered the medical school of the University of Chile in Santiago in 1970 after having obtained the highest marks in the university admission test. She later said that she took up medicine because it was 'a concrete way of helping people cope with pain and a way to contribute to improve health in Chile'.

When Augusto Pinochet came to power in 1973, Air General Bachelet refused exile and as he was an officer disobeying an order from the president, he was charged with treason. Imprisoned, he suffered a daily ritual of torture until he suffered a heart attack in March 1974 and died while still incarcerated. A year later Michelle Bachet and her mother were arrested, admitted to a detention centre, separated and submitted to interrogation and torture. It seemed to be a mindless act, for later in the year mother and daughter were exiled to Australia.

Their stay was only brief, for in May 1975 the Bachelets moved to Germany and Michelle began to work in a communal clinic. She married another Chilean exile in 1977, had a child the following year and recommenced her medical studies in September 1978 at Humboldt University in Berlin. Five months later the unpredictable political regime permitted her return to Chile and she resumed her studies at her old medical school in 1979. Time spent training at Humboldt counted for nothing in Santiago and she had to repeat the year. Nonetheless she pressed on, to eventually graduate in January 1983, thirteen years after she had started the fragmented course.

Dr Bachelet went on to do paediatrics and public health before working in a non-governmental organisation helping children of the tortured and missing in Santiago.

After democracy was restored in Chile in 1990 she became a consultant in the World Health Organization, had another child and worked in various health agencies in Germany, Chile and the United States.

Dr Bachelet had become politically active as a first-year student supporting the Popular Unity, but became seriously involved in the late 1980s. In March 2000 she was appointed Minister of Health by President Ricardo Lagos, who gave her the thankless task of eliminating waiting lists in the public hospital system; within 100 days she had reduced it by 90 per cent!

In 2002 Bachelet was appointed Defence Minister and in 2005 became the Socialist Party candidate for president. She failed to attain an absolute majority, but after a run-off election won with 53.5 per cent of the vote to become the country's first female elected president. In another unprecedented act, she appointed a Cabinet with equal numbers of men and women.

Dr Michelle Bachelet is a most remarkable woman who has weathered a life of setbacks, both medically and politically, which would have daunted the most dedicated man or woman. A lady of great fortitude, she never gave up, never complained and never faltered in her resolve to deservedly reach the top.

PART IV

Doctors who have been criminals

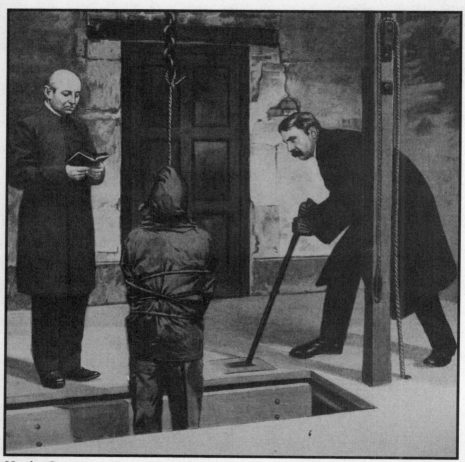

Hawley Crippen

29

Incitation to mass murder: Jean-Paul Marat and Hastings Kamuzu Banda

The two doctors reviewed in this chapter started off their medical lives as well-regarded pillars of society. They led blameless medical careers, with no hint of things to come. But later in life both became fired by a revolutionary zeal, the pursuit of which led them into criminality. They did not soil their hands personally in acts of murder in cold blood, but their actions led to the death of many innocent people of their own country.

Dr Jean-Paul Marat (1743–1796)

Once a highly regarded society doctor, Dr Jean-Paul Marat caused these deaths by his impassioned and rabble-rousing speeches during the early days of the French Revolution, which drove his fevered followers to killing excesses. For the many murders of innocent people that he initiated, he had blood on his hands.

He was born the second of seven children into a well-bred, though not well-off, family on 24 May 1743 in Boudry, near Neuchâtel, west Switzerland. He qualified in medicine in Bordeaux before working in Paris, then Holland and eventually, in the early 1770s, in London. With such a wide experience behind him, he became a highly sought-after doctor in the latter city, with a practice based in trendy Soho. He returned to France in 1777, where he wrote several scientific papers. Diseases of the eye was his special interest, and he built up a practice among the affluent middle class and aristocracy, the most famous of whom was the Comte d'Artois, afterwards to become Charles X, king of France between 1824 and 1830.

Despite earning a good living off the ills of top people, he harboured a revolutionary fire in his belly at odds with the lifestyle of the moneyed clientele who fed him. So he abandoned the comparatively leisurely life of medicine to take up politics and become a vocal and fiery advocate of the emerging Revolution. Such was the vitriol of his publications that his writings were confiscated by the French authorities. This was the beginning of a prolonged conflict between Marat and the government, and when, it is said, 6000 soldiers were looking for him, he was forced to hide in the sewers of Paris. It was here that he allegedly contracted the loathsome and mysterious skin disease that would henceforth make his life intolerable and tangentially lead to his death.

In 1790 he managed to escape back to London, where he recommenced practice. However, he returned to Paris two years later to once again take an active part in revolutionary politics, eventually emerging into the full light of public approbation by becoming a member of the National Convention. As a deputy of that body, he advocated that 'the gangrene of the aristocracy and bourgeoisie should be amputated from the State'—fiery words indeed.

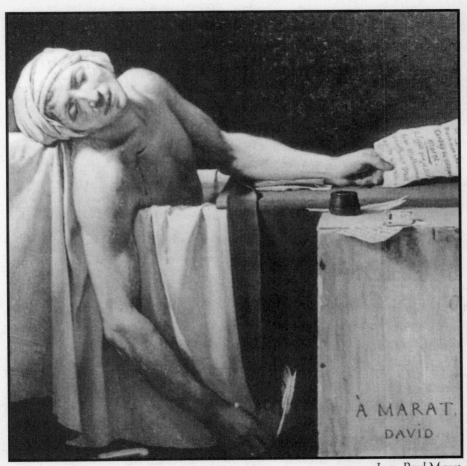

À MARAT.
DAVID

Jean-Paul Marat

Just to digress for a moment, what was this skin condition for which he became famous, and which featured prominently in his being later stabbed to death while soothing it in his bath?

No firm diagnosis has ever been made, though we know he had to spend many hours a day in a hot bath to relieve the irritation. The contemporary diagnosis was scrofula (a form of tuberculosis of the skin, usually in the neck). It has been recorded that 'a suppurating tetter ran from scrotum to perineum and maddened him with torment'. A 'tetter' is a strip of discharging infection. Apparently the skin was blistered, had open running sores and was accompanied by headaches, insomnia and insatiable thirst: sounds very unpleasant.

Thomas Carlyle, the Scottish historian, essayist and general sage (but not doctor), thought it to be syphilis. Skin lesions in secondary syphilis are well known, but would have not been relieved by bathing. Atopy, the rash commonly associated with asthma and other allergies, mainly in children, has been mentioned. Scabies comes to mind, especially in view of his subterranean habits and probably poor hygiene, but from the description it was too severe. In view of his polydipsia, or increased thirst, diabetic candidiasis (a fungal infection especially seen in the groin in some inadequately treated diabetics) is an attractive possibility, as the metabolic and dermatological disease commonly go together. But it is a bit unlikely that he had diabetes as he survived for too long with a killing disease, and for which there was then no treatment. It was too itchy for seborrheic dermatitis, though in the right place, and he was too young for pemphigoid, a severe blistering occurring in people of advanced years.

With its blisters, unremitting itch, site and disabling nature, perhaps the front-runner would be the rare but nasty skin malady, dermatitis herpetiformis. A biopsy would have been handy, but such medical investigations were in the future.

But back to his revolutionary aspirations.

At the time of his ghastly political excesses in seeking out his enemies, there lived in the northern French city of Caen 24-year-old Charlotte Corday. Horrified by his policies, she journeyed to Paris, bringing with her a knife with the object of doing-in the agitator. On 13 July 1793 she went to Marat's house on the pretext of seeking his protection and of being in the possession of a list of both moderates and his opposing Girondins living in Caen. Girondins were members of Marat's opponents from the Gironde region in south-west France. (Marat supported the opposing extremists—the Jacobins, led by Maximilien Robespierre, who initiated the French Revolution, then in its early and bloodthirsty days.)

At the time of this fateful visit, Marat was in his customary role of trying to relieve his fearful itch. He was sitting in his slipper bath with pens, ink and paper before him on a board lying across the sides of the tub. He wore a hot compress round his head, which concealed his hair: the moment has been dramatically caught in Jacques-Louis David's famous neoclassic masterpiece, *The Death of Marat*.

By dint of expressing the urgency of her mission, Charlotte Corday gained entry and submitted her list of opponents. Marat read the list, asserted that their heads would fall and started to write down the names. At this the young woman drew the knife from her cleavage, plunging it into her quarry's upper naked chest, just below the clavicle. It pierced the aorta and Jean-Paul Marat died immediately, with the half-completed blood-stained list of traitors in his hand. Jacques-Louis David has captured the moment brilliantly in his painting.

Charlotte gave herself up at once and was subsequently guillotined.

Jean-Paul Marat, already styled 'Friend of the People', was held to be a martyr and his body exhibited, together with bathtub, inkstand and bloody paper. His heart was removed and placed in an urn suspended from the ceiling of the Cordeliers Club. Twenty-one towns in France were later named after him.

Dr Hastings Kamuzu Banda (c. 1896–1997)

Hastings Banda was born in what was then called Nyasaland in British Central Africa: it is now called Malawi. He qualified in medicine, first in the United States, before taking his medical degree a second time in the United Kingdom, where he practised for several years, mainly in the north of England.

He is included here among medical criminals because his political policies, based on a fanaticism for 'change by bloodshed' in his homeland, led to the murder of very many people at his behest, in the same way that Adolf Hitler and Benito Mussolini qualify as criminals by the human carnage their actions and the orders they gave brought about.

Dr Banda was born, it is thought, in 1896, and died on 25 November 1997, which would make him 101. There is no doubt about that latter date, although the official records of his homeland give his birthdate as 14 May 1906.

He took his anglicised Christian name of Hastings after being baptised into the Church of Scotland as a baby. In 1917 he went on foot from his home country south to Johannesburg in South Africa where he worked on the gold mines for several years. While employed there he met Bishop W.T. Vernon of the African Methodist Church whom he impressed enough for the Bishop to offer to pay his tuition at a Methodist school in America, provided Banda himself could finance his own passage.

To cut a long story short he did travel to America, and studied in turn in Ohio, Indiana and Chicago to major at the latter in history in 1931. He then studied medicine in Tennessee, graduating in 1937. He wished to practise in the United Kingdom, but gaining entry onto the British register necessitated gaining a degree there also. So Banda moved again and attended the School of Medicine of the Royal College of Physicians and Surgeons in Edinburgh. This time he was financed by the Nyasaland Government on the understanding that he would return home to practise after graduation. He did not return immediately on his qualification in 1941, but enrolled in the School of Tropical Medicine and Hygiene in Liverpool, whereupon his government terminated the financial contract.

Between 1942 and 1945 he worked as a general practitioner in North Shields in the north-east of England, then moved to Harlesden, a north London suburb. It is said that he did not return home for fear that his reasonably good wage would be consumed by his extended family.

Obviously an enterprising and thoughtful man, it was while he was in the London area that he met up with politically active fellow countrymen and began to take a more active interest in the political situation of his country of birth. He became strongly opposed to the efforts of the premier of Southern Rhodesia as it was then known—Sir Roy Welensky, a white man who wanted to form a federation between Southern and Northern Rhodesia and Nyasaland. Banda saw this as creating further deprivation of rights for the Nyasaland blacks and became actively and vocally opposed to the idea. Notwithstanding this kind of antagonism from home and afar, the federation was indeed formed in 1953.

Local outraged black people knew of Banda's strong and eloquent opposition to such a move and pleaded with him to return home and lead revolt. So on 6 July 1958, after an absence of about 42 years, he did so, and in August was acclaimed the leader of the Nyasaland African Congress.

Dr Hastings Banda toured the country urging citizens to join the opposing party. He was forthright and bellicose in his pronouncements and was received enthusiastically. By February 1959 Rhodesian troops were flown in to deal with the resulting violence and deaths Banda's vitriol had provoked. The result was that on 3 March Banda, along with hundreds of other Africans, were seized and imprisoned in Southern Rhodesia. He and others were charged for organising a plot to assassinate first the Governor, followed by the Chief Secretary, then all the top brass downwards in strict order of precedence. It was alleged that the grand finale of the murderous plan, led by Hastings Banda, was the massacre of all Europeans and the mutilation of their children.

According to the evidence of police informers, the plan was that the conspirators 'should then retreat to the bush until such times as things had quietened down'. With a world history of such heinous crimes against humanity during the last century, it is extremely doubtful that things would have ever 'quietened down'.

With Banda in British custody (Nyasaland still, of course, being a British Protectorate), a Commission of Enquiry with Justice Patrick Devlin as Chairman was set up in Britain to hear all these charges against the doctor and his followers. It was hoped the Commission would bring to bear some common sense, calm judgement and cool authority to the accusations. It did, concluding that, though violence and murder of a sporadic sort was contemplated and had occurred, the reported plot was mainly 'an emanation of the overheated imagination which seems so easily to infect informers to the Special Branch [of the police]'. Though some murders had occurred, these informers had branded Hastings Banda as a mass murderer whose gross actions had simply been thwarted by a timely period in the slammer.

A purported uprising in a British Protectorate was a hot political issue in Britain, so despite what would seem to have been a sensible verdict, the British Government was displeased with the Devlin Commission's report. Their opinion was that Banda had enacted a revolutionary-cum-terrorist act, so it was decided to try to overturn the findings.

So, while Banda languished in a verminous prison, the British Government instructed the Attorney-General, Sir Reginald Manningham-Buller, to demolish the reasons for the judgement. He did this adroitly in the House of Commons, submitting that 'the findings were so far against the weight of evidence as to override the Commission's disbelief of the police informers and their acceptance of Dr Banda's denials'. This political appeal for a guilty verdict succeeded, despite the fact that the four members of the Devlin Commission were highly experienced and included a judge, a former governor of another African Protectorate, an Oxford historian and the Lord Provost of Perth, Scotland, none of whom were likely to be overcome by Dr Banda's blandishments.

The outcome was that the Commission's finding was rejected and the putative mass murderer and former general practitioner was jailed as a criminal.

But about a year later in April 1960 there were further tedious arguments which resulted in a change of political will and Dr Banda was released from prison—criminal or not. Thereafter, like many of his peers in a vanishing British Empire, his onward march to becoming his country's president would proceed unimpeded.

On 1 February 1963 Nyasaland left the Central African Federation and on 6 July 1964 became the independent state of Malawi, with Dr Banda as the de facto president.

The name Malawi had been chosen by the doctor himself for the simple reason that he liked its mellifluous sound and the satisfying appearance of the word.

On 6 July 1966 Malawi became a republic and Dr Banda was elected the country's first true president for a five-year term: he was the only candidate. In 1971 he was declared president for life.

But there was to be a downside to the cosy arrangement. Once established in his country he engendered a 'cult of personality'. All business buildings were required to have his picture on the wall, and no clocks or posters could be higher than his likeness. Men could be forced to have a haircut if their hair was considered too long, there was a strict dress code, and kissing in public was banned. During his presidency, by methods unknown, Banda is believed to have accumulated US$320 million in personal wealth. However, after a referendum, in 1993 Banda's one-party state was dismantled and he was stripped of his title.

Banda had a persuasive manner and was an inspirational speaker, and his forthright views led his followers to acts of slaughter. He was, moreover, unrepentant about his association with murder.

Dr Hastings Banda died in hospital on 25 November 1997 from complications of pneumonia. He was originally buried in a humble, weed-covered grave, but as time went by claims that he was power-crazed and a mass murderer seemed largely to have been forgotten; recently his body has been transferred to a magnificent mausoleum and the country's principal airport named after him.

Even though they were both associated with death en masse in tragic circumstances, Jean-Paul Marat and Hastings Banda seem to have had during their medical practice days a spark of feeling for their fellow men and women. They may have lost their way, but I like to think that the compassion and caring attitude learned at medical school did play at least some part in their lives.

30

Flawed anatomist and criminal: Robert Knox

A small article tucked away in a local Western Australian publication caught my eye a few years ago. The medical school was asking for bodies for dissection. Nothing precipitous, you understand; they did not need them until after the actual death of the owner. As this requirement has not always been the case, I thought it might be diverting to look at such things in times past, and where the students back then got their material.

In ancient times human dissection after death was expressly forbidden for religious reasons. This restriction delayed accurate advances in medical expertise for millennia—until, in fact, 1540 AD. That year, Andreas Vesalius—who, though still only in his twenties, was already Professor of Surgery and Anatomy at Padua, the famed university town near Venice—defied this restricting convention to become the first to do the heretical deed. His objective was to further learning, not to satisfy an idle curiosity.

In the very same year, Henry VIII allowed that surgeons in England were somehow more worthy than their then professional associates, barbers, and awarded them two executed criminals a year for dissection. A little niggardly for such sanguinary times, one would have thought.

Subsequently, the gallows were a rich source of raw material, and two centuries later they gave William Hunter the chance to set up his School of Anatomy in Great Windmill Street, London. Today, if you can drag yourself away from the strip shows down this side street off Shaftesbury Avenue, you will see a plaque high on the wall of the original site of the school, now the Lyric Theatre, commemorating the anatomy school's location.

In Edinburgh the students, eager as ever, could sometimes be a little previous in getting the criminals off the gibbet. One poor unfortunate came round during an unseemly post-drop scramble and lived on for years as Half-Hangit Maggie.

Having now arrived in Edinburgh let's look at medicine's most famous accumulators of bodies. For it was here that the redoubtable Thomas Burke and William Hare conducted their grisly and dubious business activities to provide fresh bodies for the medical school.

In 1826 there had succeeded to the Chair of Anatomy in Edinburgh an inspirational teacher, born orator and veteran Waterloo military surgeon, Dr Robert Knox (1791–1862). Such was his charisma that within a couple of years his class numbered over 500, comprising not just medical students but lawyers, artists and gentlemen with time on their hands. As all wanted a piece of the action, bodies came to be in short supply.

Knox loved his job, especially the adoration it generated, but he had a logistical problem: he needed the meat. So he enlisted the aid of several sportive students as well as a number of devious men-about-town to supply bodies, no questions asked.

On the night of 29 November 1827 two new suppliers brought Dr Knox an old man in a sack; he paid out £7 10 shillings for the body. Let me hasten to add that the man was dead all right, and from natural causes too. He had been, in fact, an army pensioner who had died at the lodging house of the vendors, Messrs Hare and Burke. Hare owed his landlord £4, and fellow lodger Burke had the sublime idea that cash may be turned over from this grave situation by selling the old man to Knox.

It was the work of a moment to crack open the coffin, pop the corpse back in bed, fill the empty box with the appropriate weight in tanner's bark, and then let in the pitifully few mourners to wring their hands and squeeze out the odd tear. Doubtless, none keened with greater vigour or managed more snivels than the two villains themselves.

Although to these two layabouts it may have seemed a mortal sin to let something rot underground when it could be sold for £7 10 shillings on top of the ground, dead bodies were not in steady and guaranteed supply. They had a merchandise-flow problem, so they decided to create their own product.

The first candidate to present was a miller who also lived in the house. He was ill anyway, so no qualms were felt over his suffocation, for the negotiated fee of £10.

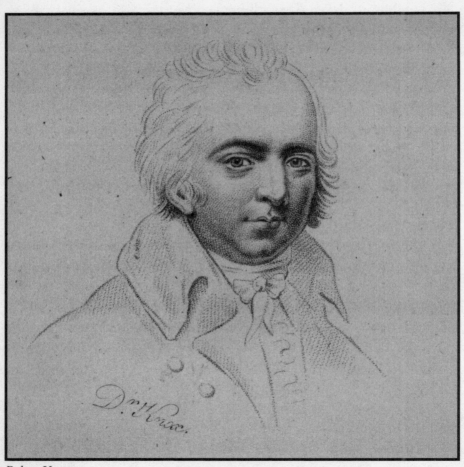

Robert Knox

Next a passing beggar woman was invited in, filled with whiskey, strangled, nailed up in a tea chest and delivered to the good doctor. He was delighted with the freshness of the goods.

The fee was the same for each, but, as with all businesses, there were expenses; alcohol and a box, for instance. So the carve-up of profits was less. I wonder if the Taxation Commissioner would have been sympathetic to an expenses claim?

Two more unfortunates met similar fates. A prostitute, Mary Patterson, was met by Burke in a tavern, taken home to breakfast, filled with whiskey, dispatched before lunch and delivered in the afternoon. Her unforeseen appearance gave one of Knox's students a nasty turn as he had known her professionally shortly before—in her profession, not his. This was young William Fergusson, later to become Sir William Fergusson, Sergeant-Surgeon to Queen Victoria herself, no less. Doubtless he kept this bit of intelligence from Her Majesty; she would not have been amused.

Burke became so bold he even relieved two policemen of a drunken woman on the pretext that he knew where she lived and would conduct her home. The lads were honing their arcane skill into an art form.

The pair had a rewarding day at the end of June 1828. An old lady and her grandson were dispatched, but on the way to Knox's establishment their horse collapsed between the shafts of its cart: they collected a goodly sum from both the medical school and the knacker's yard.

When their luck at last ran out, their stock in trade had garnered between fifteen and 32 unsuspecting and usually impoverished down-and-outs. The exact figure is unknown.

Their spree came to an end after nine months when two other lodgers at the infamous boarding house grassed on them. The police found the last of the macabre line in Dr Knox's cellar. Burke and Hare were arrested and charged with murder. Not charged was the man who, in the context of this book, is our primary interest, Robert Knox. By not questioning the source of the material—most of which was still warm—he was clearly culpable of complicity. It made him a medical criminal.

The trial of the body-snatchers themselves started at 10 a.m. on the morning of Christmas Eve 1828 and continued non-stop until 9.30 on Christmas morning when Burke was found guilty. Hare, of course, would have suffered a similar fate had he not turned King's evidence, received a reprieve and thus managed to slip through the judicial system.

The judge had no hesitation in passing a sentence of death; his only agony was to decide whether Burke's body should hang in chains or his skeleton be preserved as a ghoulish warning to other like-minded villains. In the event, and fittingly, the corpse was taken for dissection.

The execution itself was carried out publicly before a morbidly curious and vocal audience who were prepared to pay anything between five and 20 shillings for a window seat. It was estimated that 25,000 people attended what was obviously a gala event. As the bow string tightened, a shout went up for Knox to follow on the gibbet.

The anatomist was a little hurt at the imprecations being flung at him, considering it not to be within his academic duty to question the origins of still-warm specimens. Thus stung, Robert Knox himself appointed a hand-picked committee of 'Scottish noblemen and gentry', as contemporary reports had it, to examine his alleged implication in the crimes. The subsequent whitewash job buttered no parsnips as far as the canny citizens of Auld Reekie were concerned and his reputation was severely tarnished.

So who was this offended, piqued and flawed doctor, Robert Knox?

Professor Knox was born in 1791 and studied medicine in Edinburgh. He was a surgeon at Waterloo, then went to South Africa for three years and returned to his home town in 1822 to become first a lecturer in anatomy, then occupier of the professorial chair.

Rather like his famous similarly named fellow countryman, the sixteenth-century Scottish Protestant reformer John Knox (no relative), the anatomist was a forceful, declamatory speaker, and an inspirational teacher who, as I say, attracted large classes. A century later he was the subject of James Bridie's well-known play *The Anatomist*.

After the famous 1828 trial and his subsequent public vilification, Knox escaped prosecution but his classes fell away and his licence to lecture withdrawn. Though a hounded and dispirited man, it took until 1842 for Knox to eventually leave town to live in London, impoverished and vilified.

There he became interested in a new discipline, ethnology—that branch of science which deals with races and peoples, their origins and characteristics. Though in the pre-Darwinian era, ethnologists argued that despite apparent diversity, the 'races' of man had a common origin. Their argument was based on cultural rather than biological evidence, pointing out the broad similarity between linguistics, political organisation and religions.

Drawing on his anatomical observations in South Africa, Robert Knox would have none of this: polygenism was his view. With their diverse biological characteristics he believed in the distinct and immutable diversity of races and contended that 'fair races' were superior to 'dark races'. Indeed he went so far as to aver that only certain races fell within the human species! He was on very dangerous ground here, but in the mid-nineteenth century you could say things like that. Explorations into the 'Dark Continent' were at their height then, but Knox was deeply opposed to any mooted colonisation, which he regarded as the exploitation of the weak by the strong and premeditated robbery glossed over by religious pretence. He thought it was bound to fail through the dual influences of climate and interbreeding.

In 1850 Knox wrote a book on the subject, *The Races of Man*. In it he cited the case of Australia: although colonisation there appeared to be flourishing, he thought that if immigration was halted and reproduction thrown entirely on those already there, life would degenerate, and the colonists would become exhausted and eventually extinct.

He was wrong, of course, but why should an intelligent man with a trained scientific mind hold such pessimistic and, to our eyes, outlandish opinions?

His bitterness after being victimised by the citizens of Edinburgh may have contributed, but it is more likely that he drew on his considerable knowledge of comparative anatomy to measure what he saw as lesser aesthetic and cultural standards in others. He felt they failed to reveal any sense of purpose or continuity on which he could base a continuum of the history of humankind. The essential characteristics of most races were arrogance, aggression and an urge to destroy other forms of life. He thought other races were heading towards extinction.

The fear of racial degeneration by interbreeding was shared by many of Knox's contemporaries and prompted legislation against intermarriage in some colonies. However, the drive for colonialist expansion and conquest was the national ethos and his views did not hold sway in high places.

Dispirited again by rejection, Knox moved from the fashionable West End of London into the relative obscurity of Hackney, where he set up a general practice specialising in obstetrics. He was well liked in this role, not least because he means-tested his patients and many impecunious women paid nothing at all for his services. So it appears he did have a social conscience in there somewhere.

In 1856 an admirer, William Marsden, founder of the London Cancer Hospital, offered him a job as pathological anatomy lecturer in his hospital. The former professor worked there in comparative obscurity until his death in 1862.

Though possessing a brilliant medical mind, Robert Knox was dogged by notoriety rather than success. It ruined him financially and professionally, but his biological theory of race, which to us seems not just politically incorrect but quite grotesque, was accepted until well into the twentieth century. It spawned eugenics and 'racial hygiene' movements and is an unpleasant illustration of the power of 'scientific' explanation to validate a particular set of prejudices. Did it make him a criminal? No, just deluded: his earlier history had enough of the criminal element in it to give him a place in this chapter.

There were several sequels to the sordid Burke and Hare episode. The most far reaching was that the government was compelled to tighten regulations regarding matters such as medical dissection by passing the Anatomy Act in 1832.

Burke gained dubious posthumous glory by having his name pass into the language—to 'burke', meaning to kill secretly by suffocation or strangulation, or to hush up. While I cannot recall ever having heard the verb used in my life, as a medical student I did listen with awe to a lecture by one of Robert Knox's successors, and I am still grateful to the person who, in full knowledge of the implications, agreed to supply his body for me and my colleagues to dissect after his death. Truth to tell, I was always a mite disappointed it had not been 'burked' at dead of night, but had arrived in the dissecting room by legitimate and perfectly legal means.

It is a source of some regret to us oldies in the profession that the dissection of real bodies by undergraduates has now been largely abandoned in medical schools all over the world. Such anatomical training is now undertaken by the use of computerised images or by viewing prepared specimens dissected by senior staff members.

Many years later another postscript to the Burke and Hare story emerged. In 1986 Professor Matthew Kaufman was appointed to the Chair of Anatomy at Edinburgh, and during his early explorations of the rambling department he came across a hitherto forgotten collection of about 300 plaster death masks. They had been bought by the anatomy unit from the Edinburgh Phrenological Society (who else) over a hundred years previously and promptly forgotten.

Besides the likeness of composer Felix Mendelssohn, John Keats, Sir Isaac Newton and Dr Samuel Johnson, among them was the cast of Thomas Burke's head. Although he appears to have been somewhat out of his league, I dare say that at the time of his death he was better known to the public at large than any of the other artistic or intellectual giants in the collection, and came to be immortalised in his own macabre way.

31

Murder on campus: Professor John Webster

Professor John Webster (1793–1850) is unique among any collection of medical criminals in that, firstly, as a medical man, he killed another doctor, and, secondly, he did the deed by bludgeoning his subject to death rather than using poison, as has been usually the case in most other medical killings recorded here. But in common with most murderers, he made a fatal mistake, which led to his apprehension and conviction. In his case it was the fact that he failed to get rid of the most identifiable and least destructible part of the human anatomy: the teeth.

Webster was born in 1793 in Boston, Massachusetts, a city replete with well-connected families and snobbish behaviour. You may recall the short censorious poem by John Collins Bossidy, written not long after the famous incident about to be recounted and entitled 'On the Aristocracy of Harvard':

> And this is good old Boston,
> The home of the bean and the cod,
> Where the Lowells talk only to Cabots,
> And the Cabots talk only to God.

His grandfather having earned a fortune as a merchant, John Webster was no exception to this attitude.

He graduated in chemistry at Boston's famous University, Harvard, in 1811, after which he studied medicine, qualifying as a doctor in 1815. He pursued further medical studies at London's prestigious Guy's Hospital, and between 1817 and 1818 could afford to go into medical practice on São Miguel Island in the Azores. Here he met and married another American, Harriet Hickling.

Back then to Boston and into general practice. But this time he was not successful and so in 1824 he applied for and was awarded the job as a lecturer in chemistry, mineralogy and geology at Harvard. Three years later he was elevated to a professorship in the subjects: a fairly rapid rise in academic circles—he probably knew the right people.

Despite its prestige, the post paid only a modest salary—so low, in fact, that Webster found it impossible to exist in the style he thought was his due. Added to that he was a poor manager of what money he did have. So, as he tried to keep up appearances and provide lavishly for his family of wife and four daughters, by the late 1840s he became seriously indebted to a number of friends.

Among these was another doctor, Dr George Parkman, one of Boston's well-heeled luminaries, or Boston Brahmins as the famed Dean of the Harvard Medical School, Oliver Wendell Holmes Snr, called them. The Parkman family was seriously rich and were in the business of lending money for profit, and it was George who kept an eye on the debtors and reminded them none too subtly of their obligations.

George Parkman, born in 1790, had qualified in medicine at the University of Aberdeen, Scotland, and developed an interest in mental health, which he then studied at Saltpêtrière Hospital in Paris. This was under the well-remembered and revered Dr Philippe Pinel, who in 1793 famously struck off the restraining fetters that at the time bound mentally ill patients, and began to treat them as human beings.

Parkman returned to the States in 1813 and talked to the heads of the Massachusetts General Hospital about having an asylum attached to the hospital, and gave substantial monies for this philanthropic project. Though he pursued a medical career, his main income came from business dealings. He did, however, contribute to a number of worthy endeavours. Among these was a gift of land on which was subsequently built in 1846 the new Harvard Medical School. Well-heeled he may have been, but he still walked the streets to collect the interest from his debtors—too mean, it was said, to buy a horse.

And so it was that while chasing up owed money, he caught up with his debtor Professor John Webster, on what was to prove a fateful day, 23 November 1849.

The two men's business dealings went back quite a few years, Webster having first borrowed $400 from Parkman in 1842. In 1847 he gave the lender a promissory note for $2432, which represented the unpaid balance of the $400 plus a further loan he had raised later. This sum was secured by a mortgage on Webster's private property, including—crucially, as it was to turn out—a cabinet of valuable and rare mineral rocks.

The following year, still financially embarrassed, Webster borrowed still more funds from yet another friend, making over to him as collateral the self-same cabinet of minerals he had already pledged to Parkman. News of the double-deal soon spread, eventually reaching the ears of Dr George Parkman.

Not surprisingly, Parkman was enraged and a meeting was arranged forthwith between the two. It was scheduled for 1.30 p.m. on 23 November in Webster's laboratory at the new Harvard Medical School. George Parkman was seen to enter the building at 1.45 p.m. He was never seen alive again. Webster returned home at about 6 p.m. and attended a party that evening, showing no outward signs of any stress or tension.

The following day an anxious Parkman family contacted the police to report that George Parkman had been missing since lunchtime the previous day. On 25 November Webster visited Parkman's brother to say he had met the missing man on the 23rd, after having obtained yet another loan from yet another lender to pay George a debt instalment of $483. Webster said he had left shortly after the meeting, and he feared that with the cash on his person some Bostonian layabout may have assaulted, robbed and possibly murdered Parkman.

On 26 November a reward of $3000 was offered for finding George Parkman alive, and $1000 if found dead. The police also visited Webster's laboratory but found nothing to excite their curiosity.

Now the scene shifts to the janitor of the Harvard Medical School, Ephraim Littlefield, who lived with his wife in the basement of the college, right next door to Professor John Webster's laboratory. He cleaned the rooms of the staff, set up the theatres for lectures and laid out specimen jars of anatomical dissections which were to be the subject of that day's presentations. He took an interest in the workings of the medical school, and to supplement his income would obtain cadavers for dissection. But he disliked Webster and was delighted to eventually claim the reward for giving information that resulted in solving the crime. (Though Parkman was dead, Littlefield was given the full $3000 and promptly quit the job to move into comfortable retirement.)

The damning story he told was that a day or two after Parkman's disappearance, Littlefield began to notice that Webster was behaving in an odd manner, and was being questioned by him on his movements over the last few days. Furthermore, the professor had given him a turkey for his forthcoming Thanksgiving Day dinner. This was quite out of character, as in all the years the janitor had been there the two had spoken only about what was necessary for the job, and this was the first present he had ever been given.

On 28 November Littlefield noticed that the furnace in the laboratory was being well stacked with fuel by Webster—a task he always left to the janitor—and that it was burning furiously for much longer than usual. The following day was the Thanksgiving Day holiday and the school was empty. So Littlefield broke into the laboratory and entered a vault, where Webster's private toilet emptied into a pit—a spot the police had not searched earlier. Thinking that it might produce some evidence, after careful searching the persistent janitor spotted a human pelvis, dismembered thigh, a lower leg and some teeth. He also came across a pair of his employer's trousers which were heavily bloodstained. One has to admire Ephraim Littlefield's diligence.

The police were called and a check made on the specimen shelves in the lab to make sure no display specimens were missing that could have accounted for the grisly find. That done, the privy pit was carefully investigated and the four anatomical specimens were handed over to the coroner, who had already been called and was now present in the laboratory.

The coroner ordered that Webster be questioned. He was apprehended at home and denied any crime, but when told of Littlefield's find he incautiously exclaimed, 'That villain! I am a ruined man.' After his outburst, he quickly blamed the janitor, but it was all too late. A closer look at the furnace revealed a button, some coins and, importantly, a jawbone with teeth in situ. A nearby locked chest from which emanated a foul odour was forced open, revealing a headless and partially burned torso, with a thigh stuffed inside the abdominal cavity.

Mrs Parkman steeled herself to identify the body as being that of her husband, and was able to do so from skin markings on the lower torso.

Boston was buzzing with rumours and half-truths. There was reluctance among the Brahmin population to believe that one of their own could have been a murderer. Irish immigrants were blamed, as was the diligent janitor and the city's undesirables—anyone, in fact, rather than a member of their clique. In the meantime 5000 or so of the shaken population toured the crime scene, while thousands lined the streets for the funeral of Dr George Parkman on 6 December.

On 26 January 1850 Professor John Webster was indicted for murder. He himself wrote out a 196-page defence for the trial, which began on 19 March 1850 and ran for ten days. The jury visited the privy pit, the bones were described and viewed, while the defence questioned that the body was indeed Dr Parkman's.

On day three, Oliver Wendell Holmes Snr, distinguished Harvard academic, its Professor of Anatomy and regarded as the 'greatest Brahmin among them' according to the physician William Osler, took the stand. He testified that the body had been dismembered by someone with a knowledge of anatomy, and that from what he had carefully observed the greatly disfigured body 'was not dissimilar' to that of his close friend George Parkman.

A dentist then gave the damning evidence that he recognised the jawbone and false teeth found in the furnace as those of Parkman, on whom he had done dental work in November 1846. He demonstrated that the bone fitted exactly the plaster cast he had made at the time and by good fortune had retained, and that the loose teeth fitted into his plates. Leaving these virtually indestructible bits of the human anatomy on site was the most crucial mistake Professor Webster made. He should have removed them, carried them away and thrown them into Massachusetts Bay, for the evidence of the teeth's identification was conclusive.

The defence then spoke but had little to go on. Much against his attorney's advice, Webster himself took the stand, but he made no impression.

The jury retired at 8 p.m. on 30 March and was back in court with a verdict at 10.45 p.m., not even three hours later. The unanimous vote was that the accused was guilty. Later reports dramatically told how, on hearing the verdict, Professor Webster went deathly pale and slowly sank trembling into his chair.

On 1 April Judge Shaw condemned John White Webster to be hanged. A later appeal was rejected. In one last throw of the dice there was an appeal to the State Governor, the Professor doubtless hoping that his position in Bostonian society would count for something. It didn't: the Governor merely signed the death warrant.

In June, Webster wrote a confession hoping this would elicit a reprieve. He said he killed in self-defence in the heat of the moment when Parkman became aggressive over the debt and began speaking threateningly about the pledged mineral cabinet. Enraged, Webster said he seized 'whatever thing was handiest—it was a stout stick of wood—and dealt a savage blow on the side of the debt collector's head. He fell to the ground. There was no second blow. He did not move.' If the professor had hoped his confession would soften hearts, it did not happen: Governor George Briggs again remained obdurate.

So on 30 August 1850 John W. Webster was taken out to Boston's Leverett Square and publicly hanged. Apparently it took four minutes for him to die, which means that instead of the cervical vertebrae breaking and thus severing the spinal cord as happens in a well-conducted judicial hanging with a resulting virtually instantaneous death, this unfortunate prisoner was strangled and died by suffocation. After the hanging, Parkman's widow was the first contributor to a fund created for Webster's now impoverished widow and daughters.

(There was a postscript to the saga. Thirty years later on 23 November 1884, the *Boston Globe* discussed the possibility that Webster had been placed in a harness when hanged, whisked away after a simulated hanging and never actually killed, as a sailor had reportedly seen the professor alive and well in the Azores. This very far-fetched claim on very thin evidence gained no credence.)

The case generated great national and international interest. When Charles Dickens visited Boston in 1867, seventeen years after the hanging, among his requests for things to see and do was to visit the room where Dr Parkman had been murdered.

Both murderer and murdered were high-profile men and it was beyond the belief of some that such a pair could be involved in such a carry-on. It did not seem to strike them that professional men and women and the well-to-do experience the fears, joys, temper flare-ups and anxieties of the rest of us. Of course they do, and if driven far enough are as likely to commit murder as others in the community who find themselves in similar circumstances.

32

Serial poisoner: William Palmer

The name of this criminal doctor and multiple murderer, Dr William Palmer (1824–1856), may not be familiar to many people nowadays, especially in Australia, but in his time during the mid-nineteenth century his crimes were among the most notorious in the English police records. Indeed, such was the scandal his murderous ways raised, it is said that the town council in which he committed the crimes, Rugeley, wanted to change the town's name and thereby expunge the memory of 'Palmer the Poisoner' forever. There is still a rumour going about in town that the prime minister of the day was petitioned to support this change, and that he replied that he would acquiesce to their plea, but only if they would name the town after him. As, at the time, the incumbent of that top job was Lord Palmerston, not unnaturally the locals thought his name was too similar for comfort and rejected the idea. I rather think the story is apocryphal.

Our subject was also famous enough at the time to get a mention in one of Conan Doyle's Sherlock Holmes books, *The Adventure of the Speckled Band*. Further, a character in Charles Dickens' well-known novel *Bleak House*, Inspector Bucket, is reputed to be based on Charles Frederick Field, the policeman who investigated the untimely death of William Palmer's brother,

Walter Palmer, whom it was thought was killed by William for his life insurance. More of that saga later. Robert Graves' novel *They Hanged My Saintly Billy* is said to be based on a re-examination of the circumstances surrounding the Palmer case, and as recently as 1998 a film was released entitled *The Life and Crimes of William Palmer*. The wax likeness of Dr William Palmer gained immortal fame by being displayed in the Chamber of Horrors in Madame Tussauds waxworks museum in London between 1857 and 1979—an incredible 122 years.

So all in all the murderous ways of this chapter's subject, Dr William Palmer, have obviously made a deep impression on various commentators and tell of them has resonated down the last 150 years.

So who was this murdering doctor of the mid-nineteenth century, and what made him so notorious?

William Palmer was born, the sixth of seven children, on 6 August 1824 in Rugeley, a town set within the rural county of Staffordshire in the west Midlands of England. A fairly bright child, early in his life he developed the nasty habit of stealing his sister's pocket money, and coins from his mother's purse—probably the beginnings of a criminal bent that was to endure for the rest of his life. His father was a strict man who died when William was twelve. The boy went to the local free grammar school and on leaving took a job in a chemist's shop in Liverpool, a city about 100 kilometres away. With his prepubescent thieving tendencies it is perhaps not surprising that amounts of

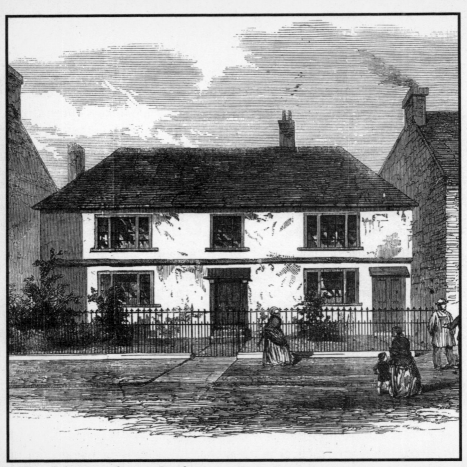

William Palmer's residence at Rugeley

cash began to disappear from the till in the shop. He was caught and it was only the fact that his mother paid back the money that saved the young man from being charged and probably sent to prison.

With his growing interest in medicine, Palmer then became apprenticed to Dr Tylecote in the nearby town of Great Hayward. Again money went missing so he absconded, this time with a young lady, Jane Widnall, in tow. Again his debts were settled by his long-suffering family, whereupon he dumped Jane and went on to become a student on the wards, or 'walking pupil' as they called it, at the Stafford Infirmary, twelve or so kilometres from his home town of Rugeley. Here a new world was opened to him; he developed an interest in poisons and their deleterious effects, a curiosity that was eventually to lead him to the gallows.

At the infirmary he became determined to succeed in becoming a doctor, a job which, among other things, would certainly allow him free access to drugs. To further his studies, Palmer went off to London and became a student at the 700-year-old teaching and medical institution, St Bartholomew's Hospital. There, and away from home influences, he lost interest in his chosen profession, did little study and occupied his time with alcohol, gambling and the pursuit of women. His work ethic became such that eventually the medical school contacted his mother to say that with her son's studying habits there was little chance of him passing any exams and she may as well withdraw him.

She knew he could do better, so after a dressing-down the steadfastly indulgent lady hired a Dr Stegall as a cramming tutor, or 'grinder' as such people were then known, to help William keep his head down. Stegall's fee was £100, a considerable sum then, but his pupil took notice of the consequences of his dilettante ways and with a new-found drive did eventually get through the course to become a Member of the Royal College of Surgeons. The snag was that Mrs Palmer never paid the tutor and he had to sue her; it was settled out of court. Questionable behaviour seems to have run in the family; perhaps William learned it at his mother's knee.

Both as a student and then later as fully fledged doctor he enjoyed betting on horses and other forms of gambling, an interest that persistently led him into debts he could not cover.

After graduation, in August 1846 he returned to his home town of Rugeley and the following year put up his brass plate outside a house in Market Street in the town centre, which he rented from Lord Lichfield, the local big landowner, for £25 a year. Many years later the house became a post office and then a shop; by 2001, with renovations it had become a well-appointed ironmonger's premises, which it remains to this day.

The new local doctor did well and was popular enough to fairly soon engage the services of an assistant, Dr Benjamin Thirlby. This cosy arrangement was very convenient for Palmer as it allowed him to pursue his addictive horseracing and gambling interests at the track itself. Inevitably debts grew and he obtained loans, supposedly with his mother's agreement for her to stand as guarantor.

In 1847 Dr Palmer married Annie Brookes at the nearby picturesque village of Abbots Bromley. In the light of subsequent events, as well as past indiscretions, Palmer must have thought it convenient from his lifestyle's point of view that Annie was a property heiress, or at least so he thought. Her father had been a well-heeled colonel in the army, but in 1834, years before the newly married couple had met, Colonel Brookes had shot himself, on account, it was said, of his wife's drinking problem.

Annie's mother remarried and was from all accounts a rather difficult woman who claimed that her drinking problem had been brought on by living with the colonel. In 1849, now called Ann Thornton, she was brought to the Palmer house in a state of delirium due to excess alcohol consumption. Twelve days later, she died, and suspicions were aroused. If Palmer thought he would gain his mother-in-law's properties after her death, he was wrong: back in 1834 the Chancery Court had ordered that as Colonel Brookes had died by his own hand his properties should be given to the colonel's heir, in his case his son, not his wife. It must have come as an unpleasant shock to Palmer when he found out that his wife was not, after all, an heiress.

The doctor and his wife had a child the following year, 1850. There were to be four more children, but all died as babies: Elizabeth, aged ten weeks in 1851, Henry aged one month in January 1852, Frank aged seven hours in

December 1853 and John in 1854. When this last child died, the family's cleaning lady, Martha Bradshaw, ran into the public house next door swearing she would never go into the Palmers' house again as the doctor 'had done away with another child'. The doctor had been upstairs with the baby when it suddenly started to scream. Rushing upstairs, Martha found baby John dead. He was four days old and had died—as indeed had his siblings—in suspicious, or certainly odd, circumstances.

Martha maintained they had all been poisoned and even related how it had been done. The doctor dipped his finger in the poison (unnamed), then in honey, and made the child suck on his finger. When pressed if she had actually seen the deed, she admitted she had not but added, 'No, but I know it in my heart to be true'. The children's father signed all the death certificates and on each had put convulsions as the cause of death.

It has been speculated that infant deaths were not uncommon then, which is true, and that Rhesus (Rh) incompatibility in the blood—an unknown syndrome then—was the cause. In such cases the first child is usually all right, but the mother is sensitised by the mixing of her blood and that of the newborn during delivery. If she is Rh negative, and her next child is the much more common Rh positive, antibodies are set up in the mother's blood. These persist for life and interact with the blood of any subsequent foetus during pregnancy, causing gross anaemia and usually death. The more children there are, the worse the condition becomes. With their father's subsequent track record, the deaths must be regarded with grave suspicion, especially as convulsions are not a feature of the Rhesus syndrome.

About three months after the death of baby John, Palmer insured his wife's life for £13,000. He only paid one premium before she died in September 1854. Two other doctors saw her in her last days and wrote the death certificate, ascribing her death to cholera: it may have been true, but her husband seemed to attract an unusual number of deaths into his household.

Though Palmer displayed much apparently genuine emotion at the funeral, he must have sought early solace after this death, for nine months after the event his housemaid bore the doctor an illegitimate child. Almost as one would by now expect, the baby died just a few months later. This child was, of course, to a different mother, so Rhesus incompatibility would be extremely unlikely, and only possible if the housemaid had had a previous child which nobody knew about.

But there was worse to follow. Not long after these dramas, William Palmer insured the life of his brother Walter for an incredible £82,000; sure enough he too perished soon after, in 1855. By now the insurance company must have had their doubts about Palmer and refused to pay. He dare not let any investigations be too probing, so in the end he settled for £14,000, still a tidy sum in the mid-nineteenth century and very handy to cover his recurrent betting debts.

Like his brother, Walter had been a drinker and gambler and had actually become bankrupt in 1849, but his wife had money, which had come to him on marriage, and so he survived and was able to follow his racetrack interest even after that setback. All this was prior to the passing of the Married Women's Property Act in 1882, before which any money the wife brought into the marriage automatically became the property of the husband.

Walter's death certificate attested his demise to be due to 'general visceral disease and apoplexy'. The term 'general visceral disease' is a bit woolly. The viscera refers to the organs within the abdominal cavity and, to be overly generous, I suppose the entry could have meant peritonitis.

By the time of Walter's death Dr William Palmer was heavily in debt and was also being blackmailed by one of his former lovers, who happened to be the daughter of a Staffordshire policeman. With his track record, the prospect of a conviction must have caused our man a few uneasy moments.

When he eventually came to trial a year or so later, several other deaths in suspicious circumstances came to light, all of them being of a sudden and mostly unexpected nature. But let us leave them and move on to the death that eventually brought Palmer to justice.

One of our subject's horseracing friends and, as it happened, also a patient, was a man called John Parsons Cook. On 13 November 1855 Cook won a large amount of money—£3000—at the Shrewsbury racetrack. He and Palmer had a celebratory dinner before returning to Rugeley. Not content with that celebration, the following day Palmer invited Cook to dinner at his house in Market Street. Very shortly after the meal Cook became violently ill with vomiting and abdominal pains, and died a few days later on 21 November. Doubtless, Palmer relieved Cook of the cash as soon as he had died.

Sudden death of this nature requires a coroner's inquest, and the suspicion generated by the host's track record of sudden deaths in his house was heightened when Palmer tried to bribe several people who may otherwise have given unflattering evidence about Cook and himself. The local newspaper carried the story that Palmer had offered a princely £10 to the postboy if he would 'upset the vehicle' that he was about to drive to the railway station, and which was carrying the receptacle containing the organs removed from John Parsons Cook at his post-mortem. Though the doctor would have known the post-mortem result, it seems to have been a very naive attempt to pervert the course of justice, and even though there was £10 for the taking, to his credit, the young lad refused.

But desperate times demand desperate measures, and as it so happened, Palmer knew the Rugeley postmaster, Samuel Cheshire, very well because he was in the habit of letting Cheshire borrow his carriage to take his wife for Sunday drives. Cheshire agreed to open the packet addressed to the coroner. (He was later to go to prison for this offence.) He then took it to Palmer, who read that the pathologist had found no poison. It is reported that on reading the news a joyous Palmer said to Cheshire, 'I am as innocent as a baby.'

The coroner, however, was not fully satisfied, as it came out during the trial proceedings that the suspect had purchased strychnine shortly before the victim's death. So it came to pass that the inquest ended with a verdict that William Palmer had wilfully murdered John Parsons Cook and he should be sent for trial. Police were dispatched to the house of the accused, but, in what sounds like the plot of a comic opera, when they arrived they found that not only was he ill in bed, but was already under house arrest by another agency for debt.

Perhaps he had absentmindedly licked his own fingers. Be that as it may, he was quickly deemed fit enough to be transported to Stafford Gaol. Feeling unwell, he was allowed to go back to bed, where he refused to eat and only took water in what was seen as an attempt at suicide. On the sixth day he was confronted by the no-nonsense prison governor, who gave him the ultimatum that unless he downed his soup he would be force-fed; he was given five minutes to make up his mind. Knowing the discomfort of having a wide-bore rubber tube forced down one's throat, not surprisingly the prisoner drank the soup, whereafter he ate the proffered meals at normal times.

The bodies of both Walter Palmer and Annie Palmer were exhumed for evidence of poison, but not enough evidence was found to charge the prisoner with their murders. So on 4 May 1856 William Palmer was taken by the deputy governor of Stafford Gaol to the Old Bailey in London for trial for the murder of John Parsons Cook. The trial was held so far away because it was felt that following so much adverse publicity and local angst Palmer would not have received a fair hearing at the Stafford Assizes. An Act of

Parliament was necessary for this switching to happen. This was forthcoming and proceedings of what the press called the 'Trial of the Century' started on 14 May 1856.

Because of the number of deaths that seemed to follow William Palmer and the fact that it involved a professional man, the race-going fraternity and 'respectable' people, the trial aroused tremendous interest not only in the United Kingdom but all over the world. About two-thirds of the evidence came from expert witnesses relating to the symptoms and consequences of strychnine ingestion. The doctor's debts were exposed and an admission of forgery aired. Tell of the death of the four children evoked horror; that of the mother-in-law produced not quite so much anguish.

Distinguished visitors jostled in the court's gallery. Over the time of the trial these included Mr Gladstone, later to become Prime Minister of Great Britain on four occasions, Earl Derby, three times prime minister and currently incumbent of the post, the Lord Mayor of London, the Duke of Cambridge, the commander of the British Army at the time and cousin to Queen Victoria, and a number of eminent doctors and jurists. Attendance seemed to have been part of the social round during that summer of 1856.

The court proceedings lasted twelve days. Despite the evidence being circumstantial, the similarity between Cook's death and that of other known strychnine victims, and the fact that Palmer had bought this poison just before Cook's death, was enough to find the accused guilty. Even Palmer admitted that the cross-examination of the prosecutor, Attorney-General Alexander Cockburn, was the key to a guilty verdict, and used a racing metaphor to describe it: 'It was the riding that did it.'

The condemned man was taken back to Stafford prison. On Friday 13 June an appeal for a reprieve (on the grounds that only circumstantial evidence had been presented) was turned down. So on Saturday 14 June 1856, after the required three Sundays which the law allowed to have passed since the conviction, Dr William Palmer suffered a public execution in front of the prison gates.

The doctor had been visited by the chaplain at 2.30 a.m. that morning. The chaplain stayed until 5 a.m. to try to coax Palmer into admitting his guilt, but the doctor steadfastly maintained that the victim had not been poisoned by strychnine. He was also to repeat this to the chaplain on the scaffold who, when he saw that guilt had been continually denied, pronounced: 'Then your blood be on your own head.'

The scaffold was in the open air, and although the execution was being held in 'flaming June' it was pouring with rain. Despite that, a crowd estimated at 30,000 to 35,000 milled outside the gate. They were mainly men, most of whom, as the alcohol flowed, roared 'murderer' or 'poisoner'. Special trains had been put on from Birmingham, even London, and a large number had walked the ten miles from Rugeley to Stafford. The execution was perceived by the local public houses to have the makings of a financial bonanza and they had stayed open all night to keep the beer flowing. This fuelled the mood of the assembled throng, and some 300 constables were needed to maintain at least some order, if not decorum.

As Dr Palmer neared the gallows, the shouts changed to 'hats off', and a hush fell on the spectators. Picking his way among the puddles, the condemned man seemed to be the least affected by the occasion. As he approached the trapdoor he is alleged to have asked hangman George Smith, 'Are you sure it's safe?' There was no struggle, no suffering, no last-minute confession—indeed, it was all over so quickly that many of the more bloodthirsty in the crowd felt they had been cheated of an anticipated spectacle and expressed their disappointment vocally. The body was left to hang for the customary hour, was gawped at, and then taken inside the prison for burial.

This was not the last public hanging in England. That dubious distinction goes to Irish Fenian bomber, Michael Barrett, who was hanged outside Newgate Prison, London, on 26 May 1868. But the notorious William Palmer was the last doctor to be hanged publicly for crimes.

Did he do all those poisonings? Almost certainly. But he was convicted on circumstantial evidence and, even though most people at the time thought 'Good riddance', he could have considered himself a tad unlucky.

33
Cora, Ethel and the telegraph wireless: Hawley Crippen

One the most famous murders and trials in the first half of the last century, certainly involving a member of the medical fraternity, was that of Dr Hawley Harvey Crippen (1862–1910). Until Dr John Bodkin Adams and Dr Harold Shipman came along in the second half of the twentieth century, Crippen was the common yardstick by which the deeds of medical criminals were measured.

This infamy may have been due to the titillating horror of a murder that involved a professional man, an attractive young woman and a wronged wife. Or the groundbreaking use of telegraph communication to catch the alleged villain. Or the hype of the tabloid press at the involvement of people who by their lifestyle and jobs were supposedly held in high esteem. Whatever the reason, the trial kept millions of people on both sides of the Atlantic agog with excited anticipation of the outcome.

Hawley Crippen was born on 11 September 1862 in the oddly named small town of Coldwater, Michigan. He studied medicine and dentistry in first Michigan and then in London in 1883. Returning to the United States he did not become a registered medical practitioner, but took up homoeopathic medicine and started working for a homoeopathic pharmaceutical company belonging to a Dr Munster.

He divorced his first wife and married Cora Turner, a mediocre theatrical singer with exaggerated aspirations to greatness who professionally went under the name of Belle Elmore. She was from New York and was then in her early thirties. Her contemporaries later described her as overbearing (which I suppose means she henpecked her husband), fond of the good things of life, such as diamonds and expensive clothes, was not afraid of boasting about her affairs and had a taste for alcohol.

In 1896 or 1900, the exact year is uncertain, the Crippens returned to London with a view to staying and furthering Cora's singing career. His US medical qualifications were not registrable in England, but he managed to eke out a living doing odd jobs. After renting several premises the couple moved to 39 Hilldrop Crescent, off Camden Road, in Holloway. It was an insalubrious area and they took in lodgers to supplement both Hawley's and Cora's chancy and irregular income. It was, however, enough for the doctor to employ a secretary.

The single pleasure that downtrodden Crippen had was the attraction he bore for this 28-year-old secretary, Ethel Clara Le Neve: the evenings may have belonged to Cora, but the afternoons belonged to Ethel. It seems Cora became aware of this philandering and threatened to leave. While Crippen may have thought this the ideal solution for his marital problems, it would have left him destitute, and so he devised another way out: murder.

On 31 January 1910 the Crippens had a party at their home. After the guests had left, Dr Crippen decided the time for the denouement had arrived: dispose of the nagging Belle and continue life with the pliant Ethel.

Later at the trial it was alleged that he stirred a slug of hydrobromide of hyoscine (from the deadly nightshade plant) into one of his wife's drinks. There has also been a suggestion that he polished her off by shooting her. Neighbours later reported hearing shouting, pleas for mercy and either a door slamming or a gun shot.

Whatever caused the final exit, the devious husband then put his medical training to good use. He took his wife's lifeless body to the cellar where he disembowelled and decapitated her, surgically removed her legs and arms, and then buried the remains of the torso under the cellar floor. Presumably, he went to all that trouble in order to create easily disposable small body parts. It may have been done in a frenzy of rage or cold hatred, but either way it was a pretty competent macabre action.

He maintained his sangfroid and the following morning returned to his normal daily routine. He told the neighbours that Cora had been suddenly called back to the US to tend a sick relative. Two months later Ethel Le Neve moved in with the doctor and started to openly wear Cora's clothes and jewels. Some of the jewellery was pawned to meet ongoing expenses, while the presence of a young lady in the house was explained away by claiming she was Cora's niece.

Later in the year Crippen told a friend, Mrs Clara Martinetti, that Cora had been taken seriously ill in America and may not live. When pressed he said he could not recall the name of the town, only that it was near San Francisco. A short time later he sent Mrs Martinetti a telegram confirming that his wife had indeed died and she had been cremated.

However, another of the Crippens' friends, Mr and Mrs Nash, became suspicious of all these very odd stories and reported them to Scotland Yard. Also it seems that at about the same time another friend of Cora's from her music-hall days informed the police of her disappearance. This was the actress Kate Williams, who was better known by her unlikely stage name, 'Vulcana'. The police responded by searching Crippen's house, but nothing was found.

Crippen was also interviewed by Chief Inspector Walter Dew, who had been involved in the famous Jack the Ripper case in 1888 and knew a thing or two about murder. During the interview the suspect used a prepared alibi, telling the Inspector that in fact he had lied about his wife's death and that she was really alive and had eloped to Chicago to be with her lover, a prize-fighter called Bruce Miller. He said the circumstances had embarrassed him and so he made up the story that Cora had died. He invited Dew to also search the house, including the cellar. Again nothing was found and the Inspector left, satisfied that the somewhat implausible story involving bizarre lifestyles was true.

Then Hawley Crippen made a crucial error.

Fearing the law was bluffing and was actually onto him, he told his lover they must move. Two days later Inspector Dew returned to clarify a couple of details and, of course, found the house empty. Immediately this aroused suspicion and he ordered a more detailed search of the house, which intuitively he insisted should include digging in the cellar. Hey presto, some charred bones—allegedly those of Cora—were found beneath the brick floor. Later the great forensic pathologist of the time, Sir Bernard Spilsbury, found traces of the poison scopolamine (hyoscine) in skin samples. Cora's head, limbs and skeleton were never found.

Dew immediately issued a warrant for the arrest of Hawley Crippen and Ethel Le Neve. This news appeared in the press, whereupon the couple decided to immediately flee the country. They holed up in Brussels and booked a passage on the Canadian Pacific steamer the SS *Montrose*, scheduled to sail from Antwerp to Quebec.

By now a fevered British and European press had the story as a daily feature, wondering aloud where the fugitives were. Crippen kept his nerve and attempted to disguise himself by shaving off his moustache and growing a beard. He also discarded his spectacles. Famously, he dressed Ethel as a boy and cut her hair into a schoolboy trim. Posing as father and son, he signed on the ship's passenger list as Mr John Robinson and Master Robinson.

The captain of the *Montrose* was Henry Kendall, an observant man whose habit was to socialise with the first-class passengers. Crippen had made a mistake by booking first class; if the pair had travelled third class the captain would probably never have given them a second glance. The captain watched the supposed father and son and could not help but notice their odd behaviour of holding hands and getting close together behind a lifeboat. Intrigued, he fell into conversation with the 'father' and noted the groove on the bridge of his nose, indicative of glasses being regularly worn, and pale skin above the upper lip, indicative of a moustache having recently been shaved off. He also noted the 'boy' was very reserved.

To satisfy his curiosity, Kendall invited the pair to dine at his table and come to his cabin to fill in a pre-arrival form. During this closer contact the hyper-observant officer was able to note that safety pins bunching up 'Master Robinson's' clothes disguised the curve of a female body. Alone later he compared features of the pair with newspaper pictures. That did it: he was convinced they were Dr Hawley Crippen and Miss Ethel Le Neve.

By happy chance the *Montrose* was one of the few pre-World War I Canadian Pacific liners fitted with the comparatively new-fangled Marconi wireless radio, so just before getting out of range of the land-based transmitters Kendall had the ship's telegraphist, Lawrence Ernest Hughes, send a wireless telegram to the British authorities—a telegram that was to become famous in the annals of crime. It read: 'Have strong suspicions that Crippen – London cellar murderer and accomplice among saloon passengers. Moustache taken off – growing beard. Accomplice dressed as a boy. Manner and build undoubtedly a girl.'

Inspector Dew was informed at once. Again by good fortune the White Star liner SS *Laurentic* was on the point of departing for Canada from the UK; Dew boarded it, but not before he had contacted the renowned Royal Canadian Mounted Police to put them in the picture.

In what was then a fourteen-day journey, the *Montrose* had a three-day start on the other ship, but the quicker *Laurentic* overtook and passed it in the mid-Atlantic. As Crippen's ship travelled down the St Lawrence River towards Quebec, Dew boarded a tugboat disguised as a pilot and left to meet the *Montrose*.

Fortunately, there was some more good luck for Dew, in that Canada at the time was a dominion within the British Empire. If Crippen, still an American citizen, had sailed into a US port, it would have taken an international arrest warrant followed by tedious extradition proceedings to bring him to trial.

Still courteous to his first-class passengers, Captain Kendall invited the unsuspecting Crippen to meet the pilots as they came aboard. As they shook hands the bogus pilot said, 'Good morning, Dr Crippen. Do you know me? I'm Chief Inspector Dew from Scotland Yard.'

Stunned, the apprehended criminal could only say, 'Thank God it's over. The suspense has been too great. I couldn't stand it any longer.' He then held up his hands for the proffered handcuffs. The fleeing pair was arrested on board the *Montrose* on 31 July 1910, exactly six months after the murder.

The lovers were taken back to England on the White Star liner SS *Megantic* to face charges in the Central Criminal Court at the Old Bailey in London. Despite his initial unguarded comments to Dew, Crippen was to maintain his innocence to the end.

The couple were tried separately and during the proceedings, the meticulous manner by which the body of Cora Crippen had been disposed of by her trained doctor husband was revealed. He had first removed the bones and limbs and burned them on the kitchen stove. The limbs were never found, but the other bones, of course, were buried in the cellar to be later found. It was a fatal error; he should have scattered them elsewhere. The soft internal organs had been dissolved in acid in the household bathtub and presumably flushed away. The lady's head had been placed in a handbag she owned and thrown overboard on a daytrip to Dieppe in northern France. Obviously it was never recovered.

Experienced though he was, Sir Bernard Spilsbury could not identify the exhumed burnt remains or even discern whether they were male or female. However, a piece of abdominal skin had escaped the blaze and by macabre, or maybe happy, chance it revealed a scar in its integument consistent with Cora's medical history of previous abdominal surgery.

Crippen's trial lasted five days, and after just 27 minutes of deliberation the jury found him guilty. Throughout the five days he had shown no remorse for his wife, only concern for his lover's reputation and wellbeing. At his request her photograph was placed in his coffin after his execution. This took place in

Pentonville Prison, London, on 28 November 1910, after the customary passage of three Sundays following the verdict, a time which is supposed to allow the prisoner to contemplate his actions and make his peace with his God.

He wrote one last letter to Ethel four days before his execution. In it he described himself and Ethel as 'two children in the great unkind world who clung to one another and gave each other courage'.

Ethel Le Neve hired some high-priced lawyers and deservedly was acquitted of any wrong-doing as far as the actual murder was concerned. After her release she changed her name to Nelson and prudently moved to Toronto, Canada. After a few years and when the dust had settled, in 1916 she moved back to England and married an accountant, Mr Stanley Smith—who, it is said, bore a remarkable physical resemblance to Hawley Crippen. She had two children, a son and daughter, but regrettably Mr Smith died at an early age and she went on living in anonymity in Croydon, London.

In June 1954 British novelist Ursula Bloom found out her identity and the two met. Ethel was then 71 and according to Bloom was petite, still pretty and grey-haired. The two remained friends until Le Neve's death in 1967 at the age of 84. During their friendship she never discussed details of the case, or betrayed her lover's trust.

The story is long, even poignant, and would seem to have been a straightforward murder on top of a lover's triangle, but over the years some doubt has been raised as to the guilt of Dr Crippen. A famous barrister of the time,

Edward Marshall Hall, thought Crippen was using his medical skill to give hyoscine to his wife as an antidepressant. (It is of little therapeutic worth as such.) Marshall Hall thought that as it was doing little good, her husband increased the dose, accidentally poisoning her, and had then panicked. It has also been suggested that it is unbelievable that the doctor should dispose of the limbs and head and then bury what remained of the torso in the cellar.

In 1981 a Mr Hugh Rhys Rankin claimed he had met Ethel Le Neve in 1930 in Australia and she had told him that Crippen murdered his wife because she had syphilis. A more startling finding cropped up in 2007, almost 100 years after the event. A Michigan State University forensic scientist, David Foran, claimed that mitochondrial DNA evidence (unknown in 1910) obtained from a slide taken from the torso found beneath the cellar floor showed the remains were not those of Cora Crippen. He had studied the DNA of matrilineal relatives for comparison. Whose body was it then? It has been floated that Crippen may have been doing abortions on the side, buried the conceptus in the cellar, and the slide sample was from such a concealment. (However, you can easily distinguish between foetal and adult bones.) The researchers explained away the scar on the skin as being incorrectly identified, due to having hair follicles which scars do not possess. However, it seems all the 'new' evidence' is drawing a very long bow.

Whether Crippen was guilty or not (and I think he was), with its gruesome culmination, its romantic twist, its bogus disguises and the fact that he was the first criminal to be caught via wireless telegraph, and was arrested on a ship by a man who had raced him across the Atlantic to do so, the case of Cora Crippen's murder by Dr Hawley Harvey Crippen has caught the attention of the public, the legal and medical professions and crime writers for a century and has become one of the great medical murders in history.

34

The Lake District murderer: Buck Ruxton

The Lake District of north-west England boasts some of the best scenery in the country. Much of the area is in Lancashire, the Red Rose county which is usually associated with grimy industrial towns such as Blackburn or Burnley, cities famous for their cotton-spinning factories such as Manchester, the great port of Liverpool and two or three seaside holiday resorts such as Blackpool, Southport and Morecombe. So it often comes as a surprise to visitors that Lancashire's glory lies in the sublime Lake District and not in the cotton mills.

Approaching the Lakes from the south you pass through the ancient and historic capital of the county, Lancaster, replete with castle, stocks and an assize court in which, still on view to the prisoner in the dock, is the shaped piece of iron that was used to brand criminals in times past. It shows the letter 'M' for Malefactor, and when heated was impressed into the back of the miscreant's hand.

In the town there is a horseshoe stuck in the middle of a crossroads which is supposed to be the very one the horse of John of Gaunt, Duke of Lancaster, son of Edward III, brother of the Black Prince, cast off in about 1370. Well, that's what the locals tell you: it is much more likely to have marked the site of the medieval horse market.

The place is worth a visit in its own right, but in 1936 it became an even more desired destination for daytrippers up from Blackpool on their way to Lake Windermere. This was because they could be driven past and gawp at the house where one of the most infamous murders in twentieth-century Britain took place. Like the later case of Dr Bodkin Adams and the slightly earlier one of Dr Crippen it involved a local general practitioner—Dr Buck Ruxton (1899–1936)—and as the story unfolded it gripped the public's imagination and sold very many newspapers.

The murder perpetrated by Ruxton was not only famous for the ferocity and nature of the crime, but also, rather like the Crippen saga, because of the innovative and new forensic techniques employed in solving it. The *modus operandi* adopted by the doctor of dismembering with clinical skill the bodies of his two victims before scattering the remains in the Scottish Lowlands led to the rather ghoulish label 'jigsaw murders' being given to the tragic case.

The full and proper name of Dr Ruxton was Buktyar Rustomji Ratanji Hakim. He was a Parsee born in what was then called Bombay, now Mumbai, on 21 March 1899. After moving to England in 1930 he changed his name by deed poll to the one we are familiar with. He qualified in medicine in Bombay and when he moved to Britain he set up as a general practitioner in a large house at 2 Dalton Square, Lancaster. In light of subsequent events, by macabre chance it was situated opposite the local police station.

314

His wife was Mrs Isabella (Belle) Van Ess. Prior to the marriage she had run a restaurant in Bombay, but in 1928 gave up both her then husband, Mr Van Ess, and her profitable business to live with Ruxton as his partner.

By 1935, the year of the killing, she had reverted to her maiden name of Kerr, and the couple had three children. She was an outgoing lady who enjoyed socialising with Lancaster's chattering classes, including other doctor's wives. The doctor himself was obsessively jealous about her lifestyle and was prone to display angry aggression towards her on its account. Not infrequently he suffered gross emotional outbursts and fits of rage that involved threats, blows and brandishing revolvers and knives. He became convinced Belle was having affairs behind his back, though there was never any evidence of infidelity brought to light later. His paranoid delusions were severe enough for the police to be called on several occasions, and for Belle to make a suicide attempt by putting her head in the gas oven. Oddly, this angry aggression often concluded with a showering of affection, regrets and a crescendo of copulation.

At the time of the murder the three children were aged six, four and two, and were looked after at the Ruxton's home by twenty-year-old Mary Rogerson, who was also to tragically feature later in the saga.

On the morning of Sunday 15 September 1935, Ruxton rushed round to the house of a dental surgeon friend, saying he had severely cut his right thumb and some fingers while using a can-opener. The laceration was nasty, with one finger cut to the bone, and the bleeding was profuse. His dentist friend seems to have thought that it was an unusually massive wound for an opener, or even a jagged tin lid, to have caused, and asked to see the offending can-opener and tin; Ruxton said that in his fury he had thrown them both away.

In fact at Dalton Square the spilled blood was such that it had soaked the doctor's shirt and suit, towels, sheets, blankets, the curtains and the stair carpet, even filtering through to the underfelt. It was splashed over the bath, hot-water geyser and was up the bathroom walls. When he went to his dentist friend Ruxton had also had taken the children to be left in his care, so the dentist did not return to see the carnage.

After having been treated, the doctor hastened home and decided to redecorate, even though it was a Sunday. This, of course, involved tearing up the stair carpet, which was grossly stained. Ruxton thought it not worth retrieving, so he bought a two-gallon tin of petrol to help burn it in the back-yard. The plan was thwarted because it started to rain. So, in a moment of thoughtless madness, he gave both the heavily bloodstained carpet and his bloody Sunday-best suit to a patient to clean. At the trial it came out that she used about 30 buckets of water and a scrubbing brush to try to expunge the blood. In the end she failed. The next day Ruxton's daily help, Mabel, washed Belle's white nightdress to remove a hand-sized blood stain.

Dr Ruxton told Mabel that his wife, together with Mary, the children's nurse, had driven south to Blackpool the previous evening to see the town's famous illuminations strung out along its seven-mile-long promenade. If you are telling lies, especially in situations like this, you have to remember what you said, which a flustered Ruxton did not, for he had already told the police that Belle had driven north to Edinburgh with her supposed lover, a young man from the town clerk's office. He also informed Mary's parents that their daughter was 'in trouble', and had gone with his wife to Edinburgh to fix the problem.

What had actually happened was that on the Sunday morning in question, in a monumental jealous rage Buck Ruxton had strangled his wife with his bare hands. It is unclear whether Mary Rogerson actually walked in and saw the dastardly deed, or if Ruxton thought she was bound to chance upon the scene. Either way she was highly likely to discover the body, so he did an encore performance, so to speak, and strangled the hapless and innocent girl as well.

Then the doctor, skilled as he was in anatomy and surgery, expertly dismembered both bodies on the stairs and in the bathroom. This, of course, was the source of all the blood; two bodies would have produced several litres of the stuff. Can-opener, indeed!

And that is where the matter lay for a couple of weeks while the popular general practitioner went on with his daily job.

Exactly two weeks later on a fine Sunday morning, a young lady, Miss Susan Haines Johnson, who was from Edinburgh and was holidaying in the village of Moffat in the Scottish Lowlands near the border between England

and Scotland, about 130 kilometres north of Lancaster, was walking over a flint bridge spanning the gully of Gardenholme Linn, a stream running into the Annan River, about two miles north of Moffat. To put it mildly, she was very disconcerted to see a human arm in the gully. Frightened, she hurried to contact the Dumfriesshire Constabulary.

They initiated a search and on looking round the immediate area of the gruesome find came across, rather incredibly, 70 pieces of butchered body parts, most wrapped in newsprint. These included a head wrapped in a copy of the now defunct *Daily Herald*. Other bits were folded within several other newspapers, including two copies of the *Daily Herald* dated 6 and 31 August that year. But most interesting of all, some pieces were wrapped in the *Sunday Graphic* and Sunday *Chronicle* dated 15 September 1935, the day the two women disappeared. Doubly unfortunate for Ruxton, the *Sunday Graphic* was a special edition featuring Morecombe's Carnival Queen, and had only been sold in the Morecombe and Lancaster district where he lived. This important lead narrowed things down quite substantially.

It did not take the police long to deduce that they had a multiple murder on their hands—there were three legs that had been skilfully surgically removed through the hip joint, and different feet and legs shared the same parcel. There was also a uterus and three breasts. Whoever had done the deed must have been in a psychotic frenzy as teeth had been knocked out and internal organs avulsed.

This was two weeks after the deaths, during which time the doctor had carried on his practice with his usual urbanity in the house-cum-surgery where he had perpetrated the felony. But patients had begun to notice unsanitary smells in the house, and observe that a fire seemed to be continually alight in the backyard. During those same two weeks, Ruxton had reported the women missing and repeatedly asked the Lancaster police to find them. When news of the Moffat charnel area surfaced, he was seemingly baffled as to why the papers linked him to the find, and in tears begged the local editors to publish a denial of any connection between him and the discovery.

The specimens were taken to Edinburgh Medical School, where the number of bodies was assessed to have been no more than two, and the then fledgling arts of fingerprint examination, the superimposition of photographs of the head over X-rays taken of it, and forensic entomology to identify the age of maggots in the specimens to give an approximate date of death were all brought into play. It was one of the first times some of these modern methods had been used in Britain. Six eminent forensic pathologists from Edinburgh and Glasgow viewed the remains and gave their expert opinions. To quote just one, Professor Sir Sydney Smith, Regius Professor of Forensic Medicine, estimated that the dismemberment and mutilation must have taken about a harrowing eight hours to complete in that Lancaster bathroom and on those stairs.

Let us digress for a moment and have a rest from the grisly account thus far. Professor Smith wrote the standard textbook on forensic medicine which as medical students was our preferred reading on the subject. We used to smile at one of his photographs, which was of a room with blood spattered all over the walls, a corpse on the floor with a knife in his back and his throat cut, furniture tumbled about the place and drawers lying pulled out and emptied, and beneath which a caption merely read: 'Death in suspicious circumstances'. Smith must have been a very canny Scot.

It did not take long for the police to trace the doctor; it was finally done through one of the children's rompers, Mary's easily identified blouse and a matching sheet for Ruxton's bed, all of which, together with the newspapers, had been used to wrap up pieces of flesh. The fiendishly clever removal of teeth, a birthmark Mary had and a bunion Belle possessed only made identification easier and not the reverse as had been the desired intent.

Dr Buck Ruxton was arrested at 7.20 a.m. on 13 October 1935, and his trial started on 2 March 1936. His defence was led by Norman Birkett KC and the prosecution by David Maxwell Fyfe and Hartley Shawcross, all very big guns in the legal profession, who were to become even more famous, as we shall see.

During the trial Ruxton became hysterical in the witness box; he was obviously a mentally disturbed man. There were numerous witnesses, and evidence of the amount of blood on the carpet and clothes was incriminating, as was the fact that the accused denied ever having been to Scotland. But on that score he had bad luck, as on the day he was disposing of the body parts in the Scottish Lowlands, he was stopped by the local police for a minor traffic infringement. No charges were laid, but a keen policeman took the car's registration number and it remained in his notebook to be trotted out at the appropriate moment as damning evidence.

Oddly enough, despite driving the bloody body parts all the way up to Moffat, when the police examined the car no signs of blood were found; presumably the parts had been too well wrapped.

For someone trying to cover up a murder the accused seemed to have made many elementary errors. His mind must have been in a turmoil; obviously, it was a job at which he had had no practice.

The case lasted eleven days and finished on 13 March, when a guilty verdict was returned. Mr Justice Singleton donned the black cap and sentenced Dr Buktyar Rustomji Ratanji Hakim to death. A petition with 10,000 signatures urging clemency was collected from the good people in the Lancaster area, mostly his admiring patients. But he was manifestly guilty and his appeal was dismissed on 27 April.

Dr Buck Ruxton was hanged at Strangeways Prison, Manchester, on 12 May 1936, concluding a case that had held the country in thrall for some months.

But there are a number of interesting bits of trivia surrounding the case.

The house itself on Dalton Square became an object of great interest, viewed and marvelled over by tourist buses en route to the Lake District. It is in the middle of a row of similar middle-class stone houses typical of the area.

On account of its notorious reputation it remained empty for many years, but was eventually gutted in the 1980s and underwent substantial renovations and is now occupied by a firm of architects. Nobody sleeps there.

The bath in which Ruxton dismembered the bodies was brought into court and used as evidence. Wondering what to do with it afterwards, the police took it to their headquarters in Preston, a town about 35 kilometres south of Lancaster, and used it as a horse trough. I am rather surprised that Madame Tussauds waxworks in London did not acquire it for their Chamber of Horrors.

The legal team for both sides were distinguished, but became even more famous later. David Maxwell Fyfe became a King's Council at the age of 34, the youngest person to have done so since the time of Charles II almost 300 years before. He later became deputy prosecutor of Nazi criminals after World War II at the Nuremburg Trials, and Lord Chancellor of England in 1954, a post that made him head of the nation's judiciary as well as Speaker of the House of Lords. Hartley Shawcross became the Attorney-General, the chief law officer in the land, and as such was the chief British prosecutor at the Nuremburg trials.

Norman Birkett had already been the lawyer for Mrs Wallis Simpson during her divorce from her husband and before she went on to marry King Edward VIII, later the Duke of Windsor. An interesting man, Birkett was well known for his eloquence and in court always spoke with immense effect. His felicitous oratory made him regarded as the best after-dinner speaker in

England, especially if cricket was involved in the proceedings. Apart from the law, his abiding interest was to preserve his beloved Lake District, and led many petitions to this effect. Remarkably, just after his death in 1962, a hitherto unnamed fell in the Lake District was named after him. After all these centuries, unnamed geographical features of the English countryside are exceedingly rare, and this was the first time in over 200 years that one had been named. It is now called Birkett Fell and is situated near the delightful Ullswater Lake.

Finally, given the intense public and media interest this murder case attracted, a popular song was adapted to suit the occasion. The song was the rather romantic ballad 'Red Sails in the Sunset', and the new scurrilous lyric—more doggerel, really—came out like this:

> Red stains on the carpet,
> Red stains on the knife,
> Oh! Dr Buck Ruxton
> You murdered your wife
>
> Then Mary she saw you
> You thought she would tell,
> So Dr Buck Ruxton
> You killed her as well.

35
How did he get away with it?
John Bodkin Adams

On 23 July 1956 occurred the death in England of a lady whose name will, I am sure, ring no bells in the mind of anyone reading this: Mrs Gertrude Hullett. But it was her unusual death with inflated doses of barbiturates, the fact that in her will she had left her doctor £1000 and a Rolls Royce car, plus tittle-tattle about the deaths of other wealthy widows in the town, and similar combustible material that the press fanned into a bonfire, which, in the end, set in motion one of the great medical murder trials of the twentieth century. Everyone had an opinion as they read the at-once grisly and titillating—not to mention biased—revelations in the daily papers. Most thought it was an open and shut case: they were wrong.

So let us follow the sequence of events and try to convince ourselves that the jury got it right and the acquittal was a case of justice served. Or was the comment made years later, after the doctor had died, the right conclusion, when Lord Hailsham said: 'As Lord Chancellor it is not my duty to comment on the guilt or otherwise of the accused, but this I do know, Dr John Bodkin Adams would have had a lot of explaining to do at the Pearly Gates.'?

John Bodkin Adams (1899–1983) was 84 when he died 25 years after his acquittal at the Old Bailey of killing one of his elderly patients, Mrs Edith Alice Morrell (not Mrs Hullett, you will note).

Balding, middle-aged Adams was a general practitioner in Eastbourne, that rather chintzy, lace-curtained seaside holiday resort on the south coast of England, and home of many wealthy retirees. He had been born in 1899 in Randalstown, County Antrim, Ireland, where his father was a jeweller. He qualified in medicine in 1922 at Queen's University, Belfast and joined a large practice at Eastbourne that same year. He prospered in his job, bought a large house in the town in 1930, and worked there for the rest of his professional life.

Eastbourne is to antique dealers, vendors of expensive cars and the like what banks were to William Morrison, America's most persistent bank robber, who, when asked why he kept robbing banks, gave the ingenuous reply, 'Well, that's where the money is.' Eastbourne was where the money was, and where money was concerned, Bodkin Adams was in his element.

Following the town's intensifying disquiet concerning Mrs Hullett's suspicious death, it was with perhaps some reluctance that the police opened enquiries about the death of another of Dr Adam's wealthy patients back in 1950, Mrs Edith Alice Morrell. Some people have long memories and for years had averred at bridge parties and the like that everything was not right about the Morrell demise. In the end even the investigating authorities smelled a rat and concluded that, everything considered, this earlier death was suspicious enough to present an even stronger case for conviction of murder by the doctor than did the more recent Hullett case. So they charged Adams with the murder of Mrs Edith Alice Morrell.

On 18 March 1957 Dr John Bodkin Adams was brought to stand trial. The alleged crime was said to have been accomplished by means of drugs given by Adams or on his instructions. During the ten months before her death, Mrs Morrell had been prescribed 165 grains of morphia and 140 grains of heroin, both derivatives of opium, both highly toxic in large doses, and both then available on prescription. In today's metric language those figures were 9900 mg of morphia (or on average about 35.5 mg per day in the period under review), and 8900 mg of heroin (about 31.8 mg a day). Sounds terrible, but spread over ten months the dose was not above the bounds of reasonableness. However, as we shall see, it was not given in such tidy and evenly spaced amounts. Moreover, the lady never became addicted with a need for increased doses.

These drugs, especially morphia, are of course pain relievers, but the odd thing was that Mrs Morrell, who had suffered from a stroke, was not in pain; she was merely a restless sleeper. Giving such drugs as sedatives is distinctly heavy-handed.

Mrs Morrell was loaded—in the financial sense, that is—and a fussy serial will-maker. In 1949 she had left Dr Adams a canteen of silver cutlery and an antique Elizabethan cupboard. After one of his reassuring and more social than medical visits, in March 1950 the doctor paid a visit to his patient's solicitor to say she wished to leave him, the doctor, her old Rolls Royce as well. The appropriate alterations were made and Adams doubtless felt that it was no less than he deserved.

In September that year Adams went on holiday. Though a normal and not unreasonable thing to do, it made the old lady very angry. She had come to rely on his frequent reassuring chats and in fact became so agitated that she cut him out as a legatee altogether. Even on holiday he must have been a man who kept his ear to the ground concerning such things, for upon hearing the news he hurried home. He placated the incensed lady and was reinstated in the will by the long-suffering lawyer. In some people's eyes, I suppose a broken holiday is worth the odd Roller, albeit, as in this instance, a 1929 model.

From 7 November until she died on the 13th, the opiate regime was greatly increased: it would seem the good doctor did not want another scare like that.

When Mrs Morrell died, Adams answered the statutory question on the cremation certificate to say that he had no known pecuniary interest in the affair. It was a patent lie; Adams later said that it was not done wickedly but to smooth the cremation arrangements, adding that relatives did not like delay at such times. When queried about the drugs he said, 'Easing the passing of a dying person is not wicked. She wanted to die. That cannot be murder.' Those three words, 'easing the passing', became the byword of the whole case, for be assured, murder is murder whether done by shooting in cold blood or snipping the slim thread of a long-time sufferer's life by means of the administration of prescription drugs.

Though there may have been some mutterings at the time, the death did not stir the even tenor of Eastbourne life. Only six years later, with questions surrounding the death of Mrs Hullett, were past innuendoes recalled and eyebrows raised.

Adams was known to the local medical brethren for two things: his use of drugs of addiction, and his regular appearance in the wills of patients. As an alternative to payment, a bauble here, a bangle there would do. Mind you, the gifted trifling mementoes were somewhat more ostentatious than that and included Bentley cars, antiques, parcels of shares and old Masters. Indeed, when the whole episode was wound up it was found that over 25 years of taking tea in a multitude of lace-curtained front parlours and patting numerous tremulous hands, the amply built Adams had become a beneficiary in no less than 132 wills. It seems he had an ability to worm his way into the confidence of the gullible and lonely elderly patients who made up the majority of his practice in the top end of town. It may have been that he went out of his way to select and enrol this type of person on his list; a list full of such people seems otherwise too good to be true.

Whatever his well-practised *modus operandi*, in the end the tangible gratitude for 'easing the passing' had included six Rollers and a steady income of

£3000 a year from willed investments, which is well over £50,000 in today's money. He seemed to regard legacies as a kind of golden handshake from the grave.

After some preliminary police investigations, on 26 November 1956 Dr John Bodkin Adams was arrested on the relatively minor charges of failure to keep a register under the Dangerous Drugs Act, false statements under the Cremation Act and forgery of National Health Services documents. He appeared before the Eastbourne magistrates and was granted bail. It was at the police station afterwards that the doctor referred to 'easing the passing'.

The police found the detainee to be cooperative, garrulous and at complete ease answering questions: he apparently felt neither pain nor remorse, just the warm glow of a job well done. His attitude at that particular moment certainly raised a few eyebrows in the police hierarchy, culminating in Dr John Bodkin Adams being charged on 19 December 1956 with the murder of Mrs Edith Alice Morrell. This time he was remanded in custody.

On 14 January 1957 committal proceedings commenced at Eastbourne, and a week later on the 23rd—two days before his 58th birthday—the prisoner was committed for trial at the Old Bailey in London; for reasons of fairness it was deemed inappropriate to hold the trial in his home town.

Such was the wide interest the case generated that the Attorney-General himself, Sir Reginald Manningham-Buller (who carried the undeserved sobriquet of Sir Bullying Manner) led the prosecution. The defence was led by Geoffrey Lawrence, then a little-known QC who was to become the hero of the trial. The formal proceedings themselves began on 18 March; they were to terminate on 9 April with an acquittal, a result that provoked widespread disbelief.

On the first day the prosecution established the quantity of drugs ordered from the dispensing chemist's records. The medicines were all dispensed by one chemist's shop, that of H.R. Browne. The law required that the prescriptions need only be kept for two years, consequently none of the original prescriptions could be produced. However, three of the firm's employees confirmed their existence by referring to a book in which the dispensing of dangerous drugs had been recorded since January 1950.

This evidence was followed by that of the four nurses who had looked after the patient at home. They attested to the large quantities of narcotics and tablets given, which had been recorded in a special book along with the times of the doctor's visits. After six years their memory seemed to be suspiciously good. They all confirmed administration had been recorded in several of these books, now long lost.

Then, as though yearning for a second coming, Lawrence said, 'If only we had those old books we could see the truth of exactly what happened night by night, day by day.' 'Yes,' said Nurse Stronach, stoutly adding, 'but you have our word for it.' Whereupon, to the ill-concealed excitement of all present, he ordered a large suitcase to be brought in. To everyone's astonishment it contained all the record books of the last eighteen months of the old lady's life, from 21 June 1949 to her death on 13 November 1950.

It was later revealed that after her death the books had been returned to Adams, who filed them away under 'M': for Morrell, of course, not Murder. They remained forgotten until a couple of days before the trial. Lawrence went through them year by year, month by month and found glaring inconsistencies in the recalled stories of the nurses, the same women who allegedly had remembered everything so clearly. Everyone was eager to hear about the last days of dear Mrs Morrell, which is why they were there in the first place. But counsel doggedly ploughed on; no plums were to be pulled from the pudding before all had finished off the cabbage.

That was on day two. On day three the defence pulled off what could be regarded as a *coup de théâtre*. Lawrence said to the nurse on the stand, 'Before I ask you to look at your notes, I just want to ask you this.' All were agog; not another suitcase, surely.

The low-key, calm lawyer then proceeded to establish that all four nurses had travelled to and from Eastbourne to the Old Bailey in London in the same railway carriage, and had discussed the case, even though two had not yet given evidence. Though clearly in contempt of court, they had correlated their stories and agreed between themselves upon what to say. What they did not know was that the man behind the newspaper in the corner of the railway carriage and who later rang Lawrence about the incident was a senior civil servant who knew his way through the legal maze regarding such matters. That, plus the notebooks, cast considerable doubt on the case for the prosecution.

But what did the notebooks show? Crucially they recorded that, first, considerably fewer drugs had been administered than had been received from the pharmacist, and, second, they had been given in therapeutically acceptable doses. It also meant that there must have been a lot of unaccounted-for ampoules and tablets rattling about in various drawers.

Then entered the prosecution's heavy artillery: Dr A.H. Douthwaite, senior physician at the prestigious Guy's Hospital, President Elect of the Royal College of Physicians, and top of his profession. He was handsome, courteous, authoritative, and had such a presence and felicitous manner that he was unkindly likened to an emissary from the Holy See. At the committal proceedings he stated that the doses then thought to have been given would kill. After the drama of the notebook contents at the trial proper, that figure was down by about a third, but the inflexible doctor resolutely went on about the opiates being unjustified and anyway would cause addiction if given in the way that then seemed to have been the routine. For the fact that addiction did not happen, he could offer no explanation.

Then, in his characteristically gentle way, Lawrence quietly slipped in the boots: 'Would not another doctor reviewing the matter be forced to a different conclusion?' Douthwaite had to admit that was so. Changing his mind, his confusion on doses, his rather eccentric and technical medical manner in his replies, as well as the apparent lack of narcotic dependence in the patient and the confusion in the nurse's notes, all introduced a strong element of doubt. What emerged was not the image of a poisoner but of a bumbling general practitioner blundering through his pharmacopoeia.

As the trial entered its third week, millions of goggle-eyed readers of a now febrile press with its front page screaming headlines, plus those in the packed courtroom gallery, waited with mounting excitement for the appearance on the stand of the bucolic and inept Dr John Bodkin Adams himself. But Geoffrey Lawrence had yet another trick up his sleeve; he elected not to call the good doctor.

For a convicted murderer not to be called to defend himself was almost without precedence in the British system of justice. Did he have something to hide; had anxiety rendered him inarticulate? What Lawrence's ploy really meant was that the harrying Manningham-Buller could not cross-examine the garrulous and unwary accused, whose helpful naiveté could well have hanged him—and not in the National Portrait Galley either. Later the judge, Justice Devlin, put it succinctly when he observed: 'To imagine such a voluntary action is an exercise to bring the word "boggle" briefly into its own.'

In the end it proved a masterstroke, and after more evidence from another medical expert, Dr J.B. Harman, who challenged much of what the hapless Douthwaite had said, the jurors did not know what was a lethal dose of morphia and what was not and whether Mrs Morrell's drowsiness was due to drugs or her medical condition or merely normal sleep. Damningly, the judge concluded 'the case for the defence to be a manifestly strong one'.

After three weeks of high drama, claim and counterclaim, the twelve impartial citizens who formed the jury deliberated for a mere 45 minutes—and to the astonishment of the legal profession, the disbelief of the medical fraternity and the bewilderment of the good folk of Eastbourne, returned a 'not guilty' verdict. A beaming John Bodkin Adams slipped away into the arms of the *Daily Express*, selling his story for £10,000.

He offered the money to his Medical Defence Union. They declined, and on his death the sum was found in banknotes in a safe deposit. Perhaps he had the grace to recognise it was 'blood money'.

The case made Geoffrey Lawrence's reputation: he had emerged from comparative obscurity and beaten the top legal brains of England. He was lionised throughout the legal fraternity and marked down for future advancement. However, it was not to be. After working at the Bar on cases that did not excite the glaring headlines evoked by the Bodkin Adams drama, eight years later he became a judge, but died within two years. A retiring and somewhat aesthetic man, he was a fine amateur musician who played in a string quartet by way of relaxation.

At first the trial did the beaming Dr Adams' general practice no harm. Indeed initially his list filled out with the names of old ladies only too willing to part with their antique silver in return for a bit of concerned listening to their woes and anxieties.

But he was harmed in the eyes of the National Health Service, who charged him with various offences regarding his prescribing habits. The outcome was that he was struck off the Medical Register in November 1957, which meant he could not practise medicine. Over the next three or four years he applied several times to have his name reinstated, but that did not come about until 1961. In September 1957 his authority to prescribe dangerous drugs was withdrawn and never restored, even after he'd made it back onto the Register.

Perhaps his most lucrative source of a steady income came from his habit of suing those newspapers whose incredulous editors could not help printing doubts about the verdict. From letters to the editor and talkback radio, however, the general public in Great Britain did not believe him to be a physician of any skill, and a large proportion thought him to be a murderer who by the sublime skill and eloquence of his counsel had been unfairly saved from the clink.

John Bodkin Adams died in 1983, aged 84. About 150 people attended his funeral at Eastbourne, and such was the interest in his life that the funeral was televised and he was given a three-column obituary plus photographs in the *Daily Telegraph*. Later a television documentary of the case was made, with Timothy West taking the part of Adams. With his death came the opportunity for the papers to libel him without fear of retribution. *The Times* referred to him as 'the classic enigma in the annals of mass killing', but the tabloids were less forgiving.

Adams left an estate of £403,000. As he had never married, it was divided among the 47 people who had supported him during his travail.

Did he deliberately hasten the passing of those in whose will he knew he appeared? Apparently not. But, like Lord Hailsham, I would love to know how he did it.

Bibliography

1 In the beginning

Guthrie, D. 1945, *A History of Medicine*, Thomas Nelson and Sons, London

Porter, R. 1997, *The Greatest Benefit to Mankind*, HarperCollins, London

Retsas, S. 2009, 'Alexander's (356–323 BC) expeditionary Medical Corps 334–323 BC', *Journal of Medical Biography*, vol. 17, no. 3, pp.165–9

PART I—DOCTORS TO ROYALTY AND NATIONAL LEADERS

2 Two royal doctors who came to a sticky end

Renault, M. 1984, *The Alexander Trilogy*, Penguin, London

Strachey, L. 2000, *Elizabeth and Essex*, Penguin, London

White, T.H. 1950, *The Age of Scandal*, Jonathan Cape, London

3 Doctors to Charles I and Charles II

Aubrey, J. 1997, *Brief Lives*, The Folio Society, London

Birch, C.A. 1979, *Names We Remember*, Ravenswood, London

Guthrie, D. 1945, *A History of Medicine*, Thomas Nelson and Sons, London

Keynes, G. 1949, *The Personality of William Harvey: The Linacre Lecture*, Cambridge University Press, Cambridge

Leavesley, J.H. 1984, *Medical Byways*, ABC Books, Sydney

Porter, R. 1997, *The Greatest Benefit to Mankind*, HarperCollins, London

——1998, *A History of England*, HarperCollins, London

4   The incompetent doctors of Mad George III

Arnold, C. 2008, *Bedlam: London and its mad*, Pocket Books, London

Frazer, A. 1969, *Mary Queen of Scots*, Weidenfeld & Nicolson, London

Leavesley, J.H. 1983, *The Common Touch*, ABC Enterprises, Sydney

MacAlpine, I. and Hunter, R. 1968, *Porphyria: A royal malady*, BMA Publications, London

Major, R.H. 1948, *Classic Descriptions of Disease*, 3rd edn, Blackwell, Oxford

Porter, R. 2002, *Madness: A brief history*, Oxford University Press, Oxford

5   Death of a prince and princess

Foreman, A. 1998, *Georgiana, Duchess of Devonshire*, HarperCollins, London

Oberst, C.R. 1984, 'The Death of Princess Charlotte of Wales: An obstetrical tragedy', paper given to the Innominate Society of Louisville (Spring)

Potts, D. and Potts, W. 1999, *Queen Victoria's Gene*, Sutton Publishing, Guernsey

6   Queen Victoria's doctors

Hibbert, C. 1979, *Victoria: A Biography*, Books for Pleasure, London

Jackson, B. (former Sergeant-Surgeon to Queen Elizabeth II), 2009, personal communication, October

Reid, M. 1987, *Ask Sir James: The life of Sir James Reid, personal physician to Queen Victoria*, Eland, London

Rennell, T. 2000, *Last Days of Glory: The death of Queen Victoria*, Viking, London

Whitfield, A.G.W. 1978, 'The last illness of the Prince Consort', *Journal of the Royal College of Physicians of London*, vol. 12, no. 1, pp. 96–102

7 Hitler's doctor

O'Donnell, J. 1978, *The Bunker*, Da Capo Press, New York

Snyder, L. 1990, *Hitler's Elite*, Hippocrene Books, New York

Wade, O. 2003, 'The treatment of a dictator', *Journal of Medical Biography*, vol. 11, no. 2, pp. 118–22

8 Stalin's doctors

Khrushchev, N.S. 1971, *Khrushchev Remembers*, Andre Deutsch, London

Payne, R. 1965, *The Rise and Fall of Stalin*, Avon Books, New York

Taylor, B.J. 1975, 'Stalin: A medical case history', *Maryland State Medical Journal*, vol. 24, no. 11, pp. 35–46

PART II—DOCTORS IN THE ARTS

9 Two early rabble-rousers: François Rabelais and Girolamo Fracastoro

Henrickson, G.L. 1934, 'The "syphilis" of Girolamo Fracastoro', *Bulletin of the History of Medicine*, vol. 2, pp. 515

Lock, S. et al. (eds) 2001, *The Oxford Illustrated Companion to Medicine*, Oxford University Press, Oxford

Major, R.H. 1945, *Classic Descriptions of Disease*, Blackwell, Oxford

Slaughter, D. 1939, 'Medicine in the life of François Rabelais', *Annals of Medical History*, vol. 1, pp. 396, 438

Swinton, W.E. 1981, 'Rabelais' coarse humour as therapy for his patients', *Canadian Medical Association Journal*, vol. 124, no. 4, pp. 500–4

Tetal, M. 1971, 'Doctor François Rabelais', *Journal of the American Medical Association*, vol. 216, no. 1, pp. 81–4

10   Sometime doctor and Irish genius: Oliver Goldsmith
Ginger, J. 1977, *The Notable Man*, Hamish Hamilton, London
Ousby, I. 1998, *The Cambridge Guide to Literature in English*, Cambridge University Press, Cambridge

11   Words most sublime: John Keats and Somerset Maugham
Banerjee, A.K. 1989, 'William Somerset Maugham: Medical student at St Thomas's 1892–1897', *Journal of the Royal Society of Medicine*, vol. 82, no. 1, pp. 44–5
——'John Keats: his medical student years at the United Hospitals of Guy's and St Thomas's 1815–1816', *Journal of the Royal Society of Medicine* vol. 82, no. 10, pp. 620–1

12   The lexicographer: Peter Roget
Emblen, D. L. 1970, *Peter Mark Roget: The word and the man*, Longman, London
Kendall, J. 2008, *The Man Who Made Lists: Love, death, madness and the creation of Roget's Thesaurus*, G.P. Putnam's Sons, London

13   Prolific essayist and poet: Oliver Wendell Holmes Snr
Parker, V. 1966, 'Oliver Wendell Holmes: Man of Medicine; Man of Letters', *Bulletin of the Medical Library Association*, vol. 54, no. 2, pp. 142–7
Tilton, E.M. 1947, *Amiable Autocrat's Biography of Dr Oliver Wendell Holmes*, Henry Schumann, New York

Bryan, C.S. 2010, '"The Greatest Brahmin among them": William Osler's (1849–1919) perspective on Oliver Wendell Holmes (1809–94)', *Journal of Medical Biography*, vol.18, no. 1, pp. 15–18.

14   A mighty Russian composer: Alexander Borodin

Cole, J.C. 1969, 'Alexander Borodin: The scientist, the musician, the man', *Journal of the American Medical Association*, vol. 208, no. 1, pp. 129–30

Konstantinov, I.E. 1998, 'The life and death of Professor Alexander P. Borodin: Surgeon, chemist, and great musician', *Surgery*, vol. 123, pp. 606–16

O'Shaughnessy, D.O. 1984, *Music and Medicine*, privately printed

15   A theatrical thespian: Sir Charles Wyndham

Anon, obituary in *The Times*, 19 January 1919

16   The nearly doctor: Francis Thompson

Breathnach, C.S. 2008, 'Francis Thompson (1859–1907): a medical truant and his troubled heart', *Journal of Medical Biography*, vol. 16, no. 1, pp. 57–62

Frewin, L. (ed.) 1962, *The Boundary Book*, Macdonald, London

——1964, *The Poetry of Cricket*, Macdonald, London

De Quincy, T. 1903, *The Confessions of an English Opium Eater*, Grant Richards, London, pp. 249–50

17   Stand up the real Sherlock Holmes: Arthur Conan Doyle

Booth, M. 2000, *A Biography of Sir Arthur Conan Doyle*, Thomas Dunne Books, London

Doyle, A.C. 1929, *Sherlock Holmes: The complete long stories*, Murray, London

18   Father of the short story: Anton Chekhov

Cohen, B. 2007, 'Anton Chekhov (1860–1904)—a 19th century physician', *Journal of Medical Biography*, vol. 15, pp. 166–73

Ober, W.B. 1973, 'Chekhov Among the Doctors', *Bulletin of New York Academy of Medicine*, vol. 49, pp. 62–76

Rayfield, D. 1997, *Anton Chekhov: A life*, Harper Collins, London

Simmons, E.J. 1962, *Chekhov: A biography*, Little Brown & Co, Boston

PART III—DOCTORS WHO HAVE BEEN ADVENTURERS, INVENTORS, ATHLETES OR POLITICIANS

19   Doctors and buccaneers

Longfield-Jones, G.M. 1992, 'Buccaneering doctors', *Medical History*, vol. 36, no. 2, pp. 187–206

Sheridan, R. 1986, 'The doctor and the buccaneer', *Journal of the History of Medicine and Allied Sciences*, vol. 41, no. 1, pp. 76–87

20   Napoleon's flying ambulances: Dominique-Jean Larrey

Guthrie, D. 1945, *A History of Medicine*, Thomas Nelson and Sons, London

Richardson, R.G. 1974, *Larrey: Surgeon to Napoleon's Imperial Guard*, John Murray, London

21 Two inventors of murderous contraptions: Joseph Guillotin and Richard Jordan Gatling

Donegan, C.F. 1900, 'Dr Guillotin—reformer and humanitarian', *Journal of the Royal Society of Medicine*, vol. 83, pp. 637–9

Wahl, P. and Toppel, D. 1971, *The Gatling Gun*, Arco Publishing, New York

Weiner, D.B. 1972, 'The Real Dr Guillotin', *Journal of the American Medical Association*, vol. 220, pp. 85–9

22 Two great explorers: Mungo Park and George Bass

Estensen, M. 2005, *The Life of George Bass*, Allen & Unwin, London

Guthrie, D. 1945, *A History of Medicine*, Thomas Nelson and Sons, London

Lock, S. et al. (eds) 2001, *The Oxford Illustrated Companion to Medicine*, Oxford University Press, Oxford

Swinton, W.E. 1977, 'Physicians as Explorers: Mungo Park, the doctor on the Niger', *CMA Journal*, vol. 117, pp. 695–7

23 'Doctor Livingstone, I presume'

Gelfand, M. 1957, *Livingstone the Doctor: His life and times*, Basil Blackwood, Oxford

Lock, S. et al. (eds) 2001, *The Oxford Illustrated Companion to Medicine*, Oxford University Press, Oxford

Magnusson, M. (ed.) 1990, *Chambers Biographical Dictionary*, Chambers Harrap, Edinburgh

24   The Grace family and other cricketers

Altham, H.S. and Swanton, E.W. 1949, *A History of Cricket*, Allen & Unwin, London

Charlesworth, R. 2009, personal communication, November

Mathew, E. (ed.) 1994, *Wisden Cricketers' Almanac*, John Wisden & Co, London, p. 1337

Midwinter, E. 1987, *The Lost Seasons 1939–45*, Methuen, London

25   Two world-beating athletes: Sir Roger Bannister and Jack Lovelock

Cameron, J. 1993, *The Artist's Way*, Pan Books, London

Colquhoun, D. (ed.) 2008, *As if Running on Air: The journals of Jack Lovelock*, Craig Potton Publishing, Wellington

Harris, N. 1964, *The Legend of Lovelock*, A.H. & A.W. Reed, Wellington

MacAuley, D. 2005, 'Profile of Roger Bannister', *Lancet*, vol. 366, no. 9489, pp. 514–15

Quercetari, R.L. 1964, *A World History of Track and Field Athletics*, Oxford University Press, Oxford

Woodfield, G. 2007, *Jack Lovelock: Athlete and doctor*, Trio Books, Wellington

26   Two rugby union players: Edward (Weary) Dunlop and David Kirk

Geddes, M. 1996, *Remembering Weary*, Viking, Ringwood

27   Education reformist: Maria Montessori

Anon. 1952, 'Maria Montessori MD: Obituary', *British Medical Journal*, vol. 4767, no. 1, p. 1085

Shampo, M.A. and Kyle, R.A. 1976, 'Maria Montessori', *Journal of the American Medical Association*, vol. 235, no. 8, p. 815

Valantine, C.W. 1952, 'Dr Maria Montessori (obituary)', *Nature*, vol. 169, pp. 992–3

28   Order, order: Doctors in politics
Encel, S. 2009, Personal communication, November

PART IV—DOCTORS WHO HAVE BEEN CRIMINALS

29   Incitation to mass murder: Jean-Paul Marat and Hastings Banda

Dotz, W. 1979, 'Jean-Paul Marat: His life, cutaneous disease and death', *American Journal of Dermapathology*, vol. 1, no. 3, pp. 247–50

MacLaurin, C. 1922, *Post Mortem*, George Doran, New York

Short, P. 1974, *Banda*, Routledge & Keenan, London

30   Flawed anatomist and criminal: Robert Knox

Gordon, R. 1983, *Great Medical Disasters*, Hutchinson, London

Collinson, S. 1990, 'Robert Knox: Anatomy of Race', *History Today*, vol. 40, pp. 44–9

31   Murder on campus: Professor John Webster

Furneaux, R. 1957, *The Medical Murderer*, Elek Books, London

Tilton, E.M. 1947, *Amiable Autocrat's Biography of Dr Oliver Wendell Holmes*, Henry Schuman, New York

32   Serial poisoner: William Palmer

Furneaux, R. 1957, *The Medical Murderer*, Elek Books, London

Leavesley, J.D. (the author's cousin) 2009, personal communication, October

Kaplan, R.M. 2009, *Medical Murder*, Allen & Unwin, Sydney

Hayhurst, A. 2008, *Staffordshire Murders*, The History Press, Stroud

33 Cora, Ethel and the telegraph wireless: Hawley Crippen

Cullen, T. 1977, *The Mild Murderer: The true story of Dr Crippen's case*, Houghton Mifflin, Boston

Gaute, J.H.H. and Robin, O. 1996, *The New Murderer's Who's Who*, Harrop Books, London

Goodman, J. (ed.) 1985, *The Crippen File*, Allison & Busby, London

34 The Lake District murderer: Buck Ruxton

Blundell, R.H. and Haswell Wilson, G. (eds) 1937, *Trial of Buck Ruxton*, Butterworth, Sydney

Furneaux, R. 1957, *The Medical Murderer*, Elek Books, London

35 How did he get away with it? John Bodkin Adams

Devlin, P. 1985, *Easing the Passing: The trial of Doctor John Bodkin Adams*, Bodley Head, London

Kaplan, R.M. 2009, *Medical Murder*, Allen & Unwin, Sydney